EVERY
MI
YE

# EVERYWOMAN'S MIDDLE YEARS

DEREK LLEWELLYN-JONES

AND

SUZANNE ABRAHAM

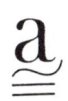

Ashwood House Medical

© Derek Llewellyn-Jones, Suzanne Abraham

First published 1992

This book is copyright. Apart from any fair dealing for the purposes of private study, research, criticism or review as permitted under the Copyright Act, no part may be reproduced, stored in a retrieval system or transmitted, in any form or by any means electronic, mechanical, photocopying, recording, or otherwise, without written permission.

National Library of Australia
Cataloguing-in-Publication data:

Llewellyn-Jones, Derek, 1923– .
  Everywoman's middle years.

Bibliography.
Includes index.
ISBN 1 875627 20 0.

1. Menopause — Popular works. 2. Middle aged women — Health and hygiene. I. Abraham, Suzanne. II. Title.

612.665

Cover and illustrations by Julia McLeish
Designed and typeset by Abb-typesetting Pty Ltd
126 Oxford Street, Collingwood, Victoria 3066
Printed by Brown Prior Anderson Pty Ltd,
5 Evans Street, Burwood, Victoria 3125
Published by Ashwood House Medical,
3/6 Hamilton Place, Mount Waverley, Victoria 3149
Correspondence to PO Box 777, Mount Waverley, Victoria 3149

# CONTENTS

| | | |
|---|---|---|
| 1 | A WOMAN'S MIDDLE YEARS | 1 |
| 2 | A WOMAN'S REPRODUCTIVE ORGANS | 4 |
| 3 | A WOMAN IN HER FORTIES | 19 |
| 4 | HEALTHY EATING IN THE MIDDLE YEARS | 32 |
| 5 | THE MENOPAUSE | 43 |
| 6 | PSYCHOLOGICAL CHANGES IN THE MENOPAUSAL YEARS | 48 |
| 7 | PHYSICAL SYMPTOMS IN THE MENOPAUSAL YEARS | 51 |
| 8 | HOW TO MANAGE THE MENOPAUSE | 57 |
| 9 | THE SIDE-EFFECTS OF HORMONAL TREATMENT | 88 |
| 10 | OSTEOPOROSIS | 94 |
| 11 | THE MIDDLE YEARS AND THE BODY SYSTEMS | 122 |
| 12 | A WOMAN'S SKIN IN HER MIDDLE YEARS | 147 |
| 13 | THE MIND IN A WOMAN'S MIDDLE YEARS | 155 |
| 14 | SEXUALITY DURING A WOMAN'S MIDDLE YEARS | 165 |
| | BIBLIOGRAPHY | 169 |
| | GLOSSARY | 173 |
| | INDEX | 175 |

# 1

# A WOMAN'S MIDDLE YEARS

In biological terms, a woman's life may be divided into three overlapping periods. The first is childhood and early adolescence, extending to about the age of 15. During this period the child's body grows and, after puberty, develops into the characteristic female shape. The changes occurring around puberty are hormonally induced, and have the function of enabling the woman to conceive and bear children. In other words, they enable her to enter the second period of her life, the reproductive years.

The reproductive years extend to about the age of 50. Between the ages of 18 to 40, ovulation and menstruation occur more or less regularly at monthly intervals, and the woman has the choice of whether or not she will try to become pregnant. From about the age of 40, subtle hormonal changes begin to occur. These changes mark the beginning of a woman's middle years, during which the most important event is the cessation of menstruation — the menopause. However, the years before the menopause and those after that event are important in terms of a woman's emotional and physical health. The years after the menopause are the third biological period of a woman's life — the postmenopausal years. A woman's middle years form a part of these years but, as a woman's life expectancy at birth is 80 years, the postmenopausal years extend beyond the middle years into that period of life when people are called 'elderly'.

A woman's middle years start at the age of 40 and continue until she is 65. It is an important and perhaps turbulent period of her life.

By the age of 40, over 85 per cent of women will have been married and most are still married or in a relatively long-term relationship. One woman in every 3 will have divorced but most will have established a new relationship. Statistically, 8 of every 10 women will have one or more children — the first having been born when the woman was aged about 24. However, over 20 per cent of women will have delayed having their first child until the woman was over the age of 30. By the time the woman has reached her 40s, most of her children will be reaching puberty or in their turbulent adolescent and young adult years.

Over half of 40 year-old women will have employment outside the home, and in a majority of instances, the woman will have chosen this to meet her own needs rather than just to increase the family income. But if she has paid employment, most women will be expected to do most (or all) the housework, and in general, to monitor most of the children's behaviour and progress. A survey conducted in Australia in 1990 showed that women who are employed in the work force spend 25 hours a week on indoor and outdoor housework, shopping and child minding, whilst men, whose wife or partner is employed in the work force spend less than 12 hours a week on these activities.

A woman approaching the age of 40 may look at her image in the mirror with increasing concern. Wrinkles have begun to appear at the corners of her eyes; her chin line is no longer so straight; she may have put on weight and there are areas of flab. Many women see this as a loss of attractiveness and wonder what their husband or partner is thinking. Is he content with his relationship? Is he lusting for a younger, more lissom woman? Is he retreating into a male world of work and sport?

The man is also growing into middle age, and in most relationships is 3 to 4 years older than the woman. But men deceive themselves. They look into the mirror and see themselves as they would wish to be. They ignore the thinning hair, the thickening face, the swelling stomach.

The woman's sexual relationships with her partner may have become ordinary, predictable, unexciting over the years or they may continue to be wonderful. Male sexual problems increase as the man enters middle age. Many men's sexual desire is beginning to decrease; they take longer to reach orgasm; and a few men find that they are developing erectile failure (impotence). Many men seek to deny that there is any change in their sexuality, or blame the change on their partner, who is perceived to be not so attractive as formerly, or not as interested in sex.

Many men blame the woman rather than recognising that their life style with too much work, too much alcohol and insufficient exercise (or too much exercise), is the reason for the change in their sexual desire and performance. If the couple cannot communicate comfortably about their sexual desires and needs, the resulting emotional upset may affect the woman more than the man.

As the menopause is perceived as a major change in life (both by many women and by many men), much of this book is about the menopausal years, but health issues in the years before the menopause and in the postmenopausal years will be discussed.

If there is to be a message for women in their middle years, it is this: the change of life is *not* the end of life and there are many years of fulfilment and excitement in the later years of a woman's life.

# 2

# A WOMAN'S REPRODUCTIVE ORGANS

Because many women in their middle years (and their partners) lack knowledge about the organs which are affected considerably during these years, it is perhaps not inappropriate to start with a description — a type of map — of a woman's genital organs. It is an odd finding, in several surveys, that many women have never looked 'down there', using a mirror. Women regularly look at other parts of their body, but their external genital organs are largely ignored. It is hoped that the next few pages will help those women who would like to know more; those who already know their anatomy, may wish to skip this chapter.

## THE EXTERNAL GENITAL ORGANS

The anatomical name for the area of the external genitalia in the female is the vulva. It is made up of several structures that surround the entrance to the vagina, each of which has its own separate function (Fig. 2.1). The labia majora (or the large lips of the vagina) are two large folds of skin, which contain sweat glands and hair follicles embedded in fat. The size of the labia majora varies considerably. In infancy and old age they are small, and the fat is not present; in the reproductive years, between puberty and the menopause, they are well filled with fatty tissue. Looked at from between the legs, they join together in the pad of fat that surmounts the pelvic bone, and was called the 'mount of Venus' (mons veneris) by the ancient anatomists, when they noted that it was most developed in the reproductive years. Both of the labia, and more particularly the mons veneris, are covered with hair, the quantity of which varies from

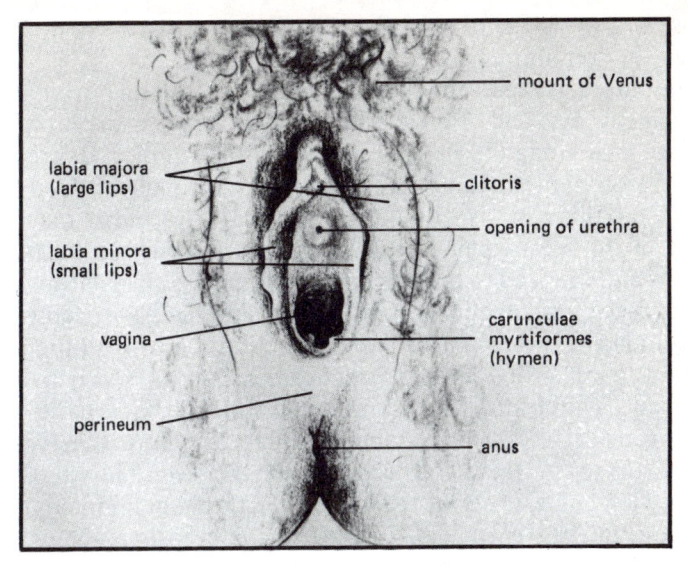

Figure 2.1: The external genitals in a woman who has had a child

woman to woman. The pubic hair on the abdominal side of the mons veneris terminates in a straight line, while in the male the hair stretches upwards in an inverted 'V' to reach the umbilicus.

The inner surfaces of the labia majora are free from hair, and are separated by a small groove from the thin labia minora, which guard the entrance to the vagina.

The labia minora (the small lips) are delicate folds of skin, which contain little fatty tissue. They vary in size, and it was once believed that large labia minora were due to masturbation, which at that time was considered evil. It is now known that this is nonsense. In front, the labia minora divide into two folds, one of which passes over, and the other under the clitoris, and at the back they join to form the fourchette, which is always torn during childbirth. In the reproductive years, the labia minora are hidden by the enlarged labia majora, but in childhood and old age the labia minora appear more prominent because the labia majora are relatively small.

The clitoris is the exact female equivalent of the male penis. The fold of the labia minora that passes over it is equivalent to the male foreskin (prepuce). It is called the 'hood' and it covers and protects the sensitive end (or glans) of the clitoris. The fold of skin that passes under the clitoris is the equivalent of the small band of tissue that joins the pink glans of the penis to the skin that covers it, and is called the frenulum.

The clitoris is made up of tissue that fills with blood during sexual excitement. The end of the clitoris is often very sensitive to touch, but the area along the shaft of the clitoris, if stimulated, produces sexual arousal in the same way that a man is sexually aroused when the shaft of his penis is stimulated. In sexual intercourse, the movement of the man's penis in the vagina indirectly stimulates the clitoris and can lead to the woman having an orgasm. Many women do not reach orgasm during sexual intercourse but have deeply satisfying orgasms if they masturbate their clitoral area with their own finger or hand, or if a sexual partner caresses the area with his finger or tongue. The clitoris varies considerably in size, but is usually that of a green pea; as sexual excitement mounts, the clitoris increases in size. Once again, this varies considerably between individuals.

The cleft below the clitoris and between the labia minora is called the vestibule (or entrance). Just below the clitoris is the external opening of that part of the urinary tract (the urethra) that connects the bladder to the outside world. In old age, the urethral orifice may stretch and the lining of the lower part of the urethra may be exposed.

Below the external orifice is the hymen, which surrounds the vaginal orifice. The hymen is a thin incomplete fold of membrane, with one or more apertures in it. It varies considerably in shape and in elasticity, but is generally stretched or torn during the first attempt at sexual intercourse. The tearing may be followed by a minute amount of bleeding. In many cultures the rupture of the hymen (also called the maidenhead) and the consequent bleed is considered a sign that the girl was a virgin at the time of marriage; the bed is inspected on the morning after the first night of the honeymoon for evidence of blood. Although an intact hymen is considered a sign of virginity, it is not a reliable sign, as in some cases sexual intercourse fails to cause a tear and in others the hymen may have been torn previously by exploring fingers, either of the girl herself or of her sexual partner. Childbirth causes a greater tearing of the hymen, and after delivery only a few tags remain. Just outside the hymen, still within the vestibule but deep beneath the skin, are two collections of erectile tissues that fill with blood during sexual arousal. Deep in the backward part of the vestibule are two pea-sized glands, which secrete fluid during sexual arousal and moisten the entrance to the vagina, so that the penis may more readily enter it without discomfort. These glands, known as Bartholin's glands, occasionally become infected.

The area of the vulva between the posterior fourchette and the anus, and the muscles that lie under the skin, form a pyramid shaped wedge of tissue separating the vagina and the rectum. It is called the perineum, and is of considerable importance in childbirth.

It is a matter of constant surprise to us that many women have never looked at their own, or any other woman's external genitals, and consequently are concerned that they may be abnormal. We would agree that the diagram on page 5 is idealized to some extent and that a considerable range of shapes and sizes of the labia minora, the hymen and the hood of the clitoris is usual; so that if a woman looks at her external genitals with a mirror and finds what she sees is not exactly like the diagram, particularly in the length and shape of the labia minora, she should not be alarmed.

This reluctance to look at one's own genitals is a feminine trait (after all, men constantly look at and touch their external genitals) and has its origin in the attitudes that many mothers gave their daughters about their genitals. These attitudes are that the external genitals are 'private', ugly, should never be touched or 'played with', have a smell, and are 'dirty'.

Such indoctrination in childhood can have sad consequences to a woman's image of her own body and in her sexual response. Even the medical word for the external genitals of a woman is negatively loaded: it is the pudendum, which derives from the Latin word pudere — 'to be ashamed'. A woman should not be ashamed of or disgusted by her external genitals and should look at them to become familiar with their unique shape.

## THE INTERNAL GENITAL ORGANS

*The vagina* This is a muscular tube that stretches upwards and backwards from the vestibule to reach the uterus. As well as being muscular, it contains a well developed network of veins, which become distended in sexual arousal. Normally the walls of the vagina lie close together, the vagina being a potential cavity, which is distended by intravaginal tampons used during menstruation, by the penis during sexual intercourse, and in childbirth, when it stretches very considerably to permit the baby to be born. The vagina is about 9 cm (3¾ in.) long and at the upper end the cervix (or neck) of the uterus projects into it (Fig. 2.2). The vagina lies between

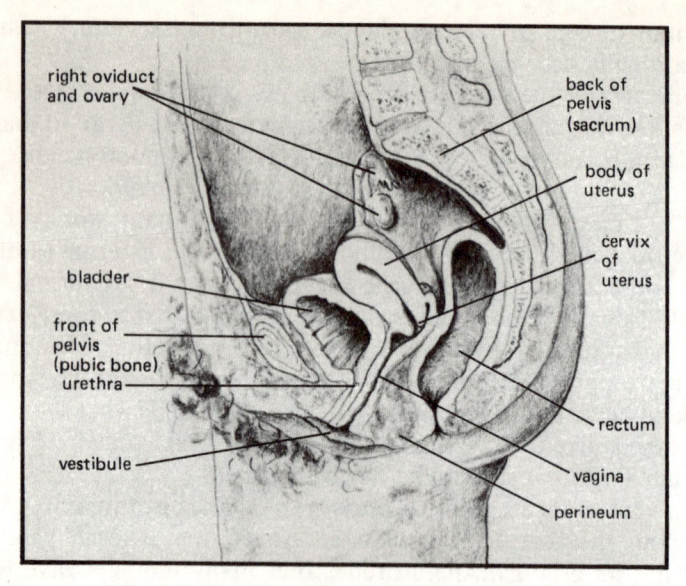

Figure 2.2: A woman's internal genital organs

the bladder in front and the rectum (or back passage) behind. At the sides it is surrounded and protected by the strong muscles of the floor of the pelvis. Unless the vagina has been damaged, injured or tightened at operation, or has not developed due to an absence of sex hormones, its size is quite adequate for sexual intercourse, and menopause usually does not influence this function. The vagina itself is a tube with an outer layer of muscle and an inner layer of cells.

The vagina, the bladder and the rectum are kept in their proper position in the pelvis by a fan-shaped muscle which stretches like a sling from each inner wall of the bony pelvis to meet in the mid line. This is called the pelvic diaphragm. The vagina, the rectum and the urethra (the tube from the bladder to the vulva), pass through 'holes' in the pelvic diaphragm to reach the vulva. Actually, they are not really holes, as the muscles of the pelvic diaphragm mingle with the muscles surrounding the organs, to keep them in place. If the muscles and the tissues of the pelvic diaphragm are weakened or stretched (as may occur during childbirth) the support is reduced and the vaginal walls may bulge downwards causing a prolapse (see page 135)

The vagina is a remarkable organ. Not only is it capable of great distension, but it keeps itself clean. The cells that form its walls are 30 cells deep, lying on each other like the bricks of a house wall. In the reproductive years, the top layer of cells is constantly being shed into the vagina, where the cells are acted upon by a small bacillus that normally lives there, to produce lactic acid. The lactic acid kills any contaminating germs that may happen to get into the vagina. Because of this, 'cleansing' vaginal douches, so popular at one time in the United States, are unnecessary. In the years after the menopause, the lining tends to become thin, and few cells are shed, so little or no lactic acid is formed and contaminating germs may grow. This sometimes results in inflammation of the vagina, particularly in elderly women.

*The uterus* The uterus is an even more remarkable organ than the vagina. In the reproductive years, when the woman is not pregnant, it is pear shaped, averages 9 cm (3¾ in.) in length, 6 cm (2½ in.) in width at its widest point and weighs 60 g (2 oz.). The uterus is a muscular organ, located in the middle of the bony pelvis, and lying between the bladder in front and the bowel behind (Fig. 2.2). Its muscular front and back walls bulge into the cavity, which is normally narrow and slit-like, unless pregnancy occurs. Viewed from in front, the cavity is triangular and is lined with a special tissue made up of glands in a network of cells. This tissue is called the endometrium and it undergoes changes during each menstrual cycle. For descriptive purposes, the uterus is divided into an upper part, or body, and a lower portion, or cervix uteri. The word cervix means neck, so that the 'cervix uteri' means the neck of the womb. The cavity is narrow in the cervix, where it is called the cervical canal, widest in the body of the uterus and then narrow again towards the cornu (or horn), where the cavity is continuous with the hollow Fallopian tube (Fig. 2.3). The cervix projects into the upper part of the vagina and is a particular place where cancer sometimes develops. The cancerous change in the cells of the cervix are preceded by alterations in their appearance, which may be seen when viewed through a microscope. If the alterations are detected, action can be taken to treat them so that cancer does not develop. This is the reason for recommending the examination of these cells by the Pap smear at regular intervals from when the woman is about 20 years old.

The lower part of the uterus and the upper part of the cervix are

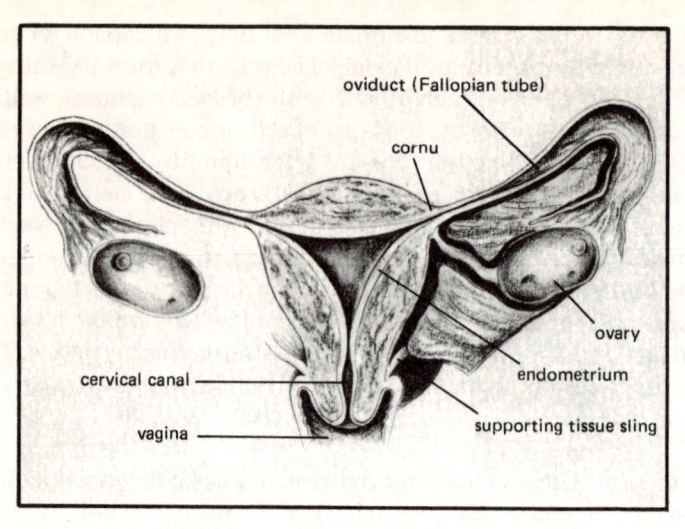

Figure 2.3: The cavity of the uterus and tubes

supported by a sling of special tissues, which stretch to the muscles of the pelvic wall in a fan-like manner. These supports may be stretched in childbirth, leading to a prolapse later in life. With better obstetrics and better education for childbirth, this complication is today much less likely to occur.

The uterus usually lies bent forward at an angle of 90° to the vagina, resting on the bladder. As the bladder fills it rotates backwards; as it empties the uterus falls forward again.

*The oviducts* The oviducts (or Fallopian tubes) are two small, hollow tubes, one on each side, which stretch for about 10 cm (4 in.) from the upper part of the uterus to lie in contact with the ovary on each side. Each tube is about the size of a drinking straw. The outer end of each oviduct is divided into long finger-like processes, and it is thought that these sweep up the egg when it is expelled from the ovary.

*The ovaries* In the reproductive years, the two ovaries are almond-shaped organs, averaging 3.5 cm (1½ in.) in length and 2 cm (¾ in.) in breadth. After the menopause, they decrease in size and in old age are less than half their adult size. Each ovary has a centre made up of small cells and a mesh of vessels. Surrounding this is the ovary proper, which contains about 200 000 egg cells lying in a cellular bed; outside this again, protecting the egg cells and the ovarian tissue, is a thickened layer of tissue. The ovaries are the equivalent of the male testes, and in addition to containing the egg cells on which all human life depends, the ovaries produce the female sex hormones during the reproductive years.

## CHANGES AFTER THE MENOPAUSE

The tissues that make up a woman's genital organs are very responsive to the female sex hormones, oestrogen and progesterone. Oestrogen, which is produced in a woman's ovaries from puberty onwards, stimulates the growth of all the genital organs. This is why following puberty a woman's vagina grows and becomes moist, the uterus grows and menstruation starts, the Fallopian tubes become longer and thicker and the ovaries increase in size. The growth effect of oestrogen is modified by progesterone and a delicate relationship exists between the two hormones.

After the menopause very little progesterone is secreted and the level of oestrogen in the blood falls by at least 50 per cent. This is because the ovaries, having lost all their follicles, cease to produce oestrogen. However, oestrogen is still produced. This occurs because chemicals from another gland in the body, the adrenal gland, are converted into oestrogen in a woman's body fat. The quantity of oestrogen varies, depending principally on the quantities of fat in her body.

Over the years following menopause, a woman's genital organs become smaller. Her ovaries shrivel, each becoming the size of a small almond, and the Fallopian tubes become thin. Her uterus becomes small, in extreme old age often becoming no bigger than a thimble. Her vagina becomes narrower and its walls thinner. This may have two effects. The first is that the woman may develop a vaginal discomfort. The second is that sexual intercourse may become painful or impossible. The woman's vulva changes in appearance. The fat in her labia majora disappears, and her labia minora become more prominent. Slowly the vulva shrivels becoming a narrow dry slit in some old women. The changes may also affect a woman's bladder and may be a factor in some women of an increasing need to pass urine, especially at night, or of bladder infection. A few postmenopausal women find that they cannot control their urine, it dribbles out unexpectedly.

These changes occur at speeds that vary between women, and are halted or slowed if a woman either produces her own supply of oestrogen or takes oestrogen tablets.

A woman's breasts also respond readily to the stimulation of oestrogen. Many women observe that their breasts become fuller and more 'knotty' in the 2 weeks before menstruation. This is due to the effects of oestrogen. After the menopause the stimulating effect diminishes and the gland tissue in the breasts is reduced. Some post-menopausal women's breasts become small; in other women they become larger as more fat is deposited in them.

## MENSTRUATION AND THE MENOPAUSE

During the reproductive years menstruation occurs regularly at reasonably predictable intervals. Most menstrual cycles, at least after the age of 16 and before the age of 45, are associated with ovulation, which occurs between 10 and 18 days before each menstruation starts whatever the length of the menstrual cycle.

Menstruation itself is the end of a complicated series of events. The ultimate controller of these events is a part of the brain called the hypothalamus, and even this part is affected by emotions and upsets. This is demonstrated by the fact that menstruation may cease after a particularly strong emotional upset. The absence of periods, which is called amenorrhoea, may persist for varying lengths of time. If the woman is not pregnant the periods usually return after 2 or 3 months; but in some women, amenorrhoea may persist for much longer. When this occurs, the woman usually visits a doctor. At this visit the doctor enquires about the woman's eating habits, her exercise patterns, and whether she has lost or gained weight. If the amenorrhoea has lasted for more than 9 months, the doctor usually takes blood to measure various hormones, as menstruation is regulated by them.

The sequence of hormonal events that precedes each monthly period is complicated and is more readily understood if one starts at the time of menstruation and traces what happens up to the time the next menstrual period occurs.

During the menstrual cycle, starting during menstruation, an area in the lowest part of the brain, the hypothalamus, releases quantities of a substance called gonadotrophin releasing hormone into the blood that supplies the pituitary gland. The hormone causes special cells in the pituitary gland to secrete a hormone called the follicle-stimulating hormone or FSH. The amount of FSH in the blood rises and stimulates the growth of 10 to 20 egg follicles. These follicles grow and as they do so they manufacture oestrogen, so that the amount of this special female sex hormone increases in the blood. Oestrogen has several effects on the tissues that make up the genital tract, but the one in which we are particularly interested is its action on the lining of the uterus. Oestrogen stimulates the lining to grow. At the end of the previous menstruation most of the lining had crumbled away and, mixed with blood and tissue fluid, had been shed as the menstrual flow. The lining is made up of narrow tubes, called endometrial glands, set in several layers of cells, called endometrial stromal cells. Oestrogen makes the glands grow, and the layers of stromal cells increase, or proliferate. Because of this, the changes in the uterus are called proliferative and this part of the cycle is called the proliferative phase of the menstrual cycle. As the follicles grow the amount of oestrogen in the blood continues to rise, and by 13 days after the onset of the previous menstruation, it has increased six-fold above the level found at the onset. The rising levels of oestrogen in the blood have an effect called a 'feed-back' on the hypothalamus, causing a change in gonadotrophin releasing hormone. The altered hormone is carried down the blood vessels that connect the hypothalamus to the pituitary gland, where certain specialized cells produce a substance called luteinizing hormone, or LH (Fig. 2.4). This hormone is so-called because it induces one of the egg follicles to burst and expel its contained egg, and it then changes the cells that make up the follicle to a bright yellow colour. (The Latin word for yellow is 'luteus' — hence the luteinizing, or yellow-making hormone). On about the 14th day after the onset of the previous menstrual period, a sudden surge of luteinizing hormone sweeps through the blood stream. It reaches the ovary, where it induces 'bursting' of the egg follicle that has grown the most, and that is blown up and tight like a tiny balloon. During growth this particular follicle had swollen and moved through the ovary to reach its surface, where it made a tiny bulge that can be seen by the naked eye. Suddenly, under the influence of the luteinizing hormone, the follicle bursts and the egg is pushed out, together with the fluid in which it lay. The egg is caught in the finger-like ends of the oviduct, which caress the ovary at this time, and is moved slowly but gently into the cavity of the oviduct tube, where fertilization takes place, if this is to happen (Fig. 2.5).

Once the egg (ovum) has been expelled, the now empty follicle collapses, and the luteinizing hormone acts on the cells of its wall,

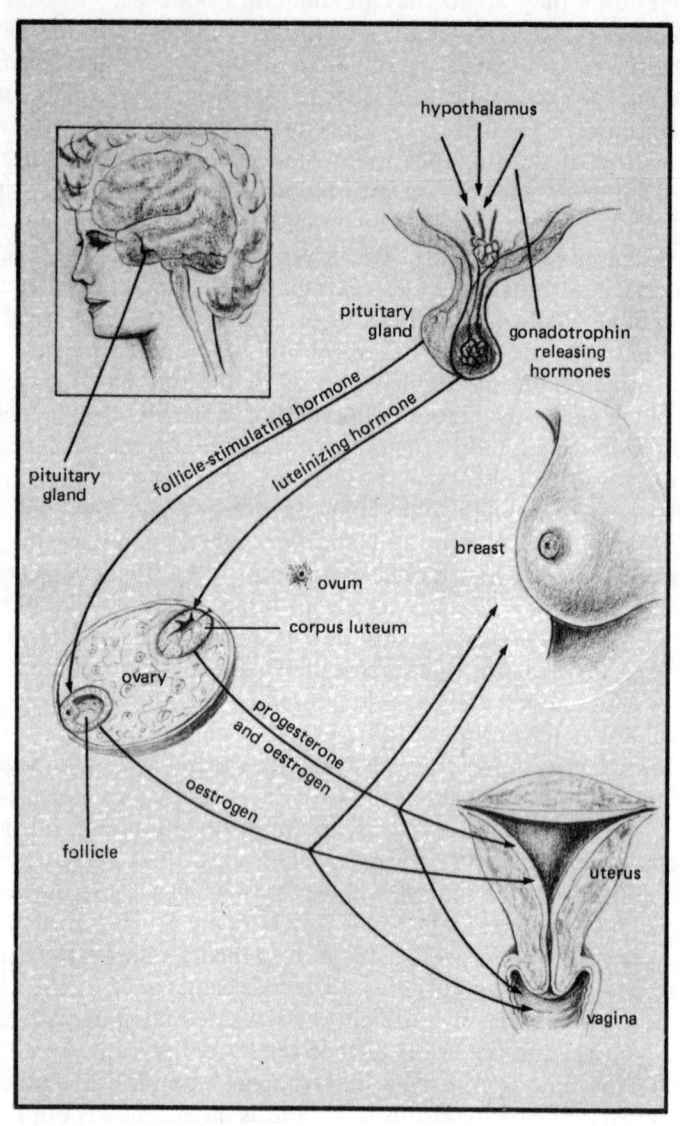

Figure 2.4: The control of menstruation

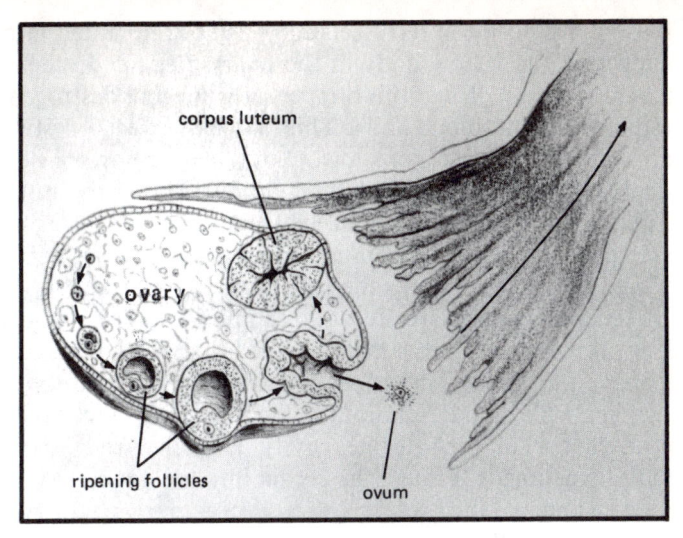

Figure 2.5: The growth of stimulated follicles in the ovary during a menstrual cycle

turning them yellow. The collapsed follicle is called a yellow body or, in Latin, a corpus luteum. The change in colour of the cells of the corpus luteum is due to a change in their activity. Now not only do they continue to secrete oestrogen (together with the other 11 to 19 stimulated follicles that failed to grow as quickly), but uniquely they also manufacture a new hormone called progesterone. The name is apt, for the hormone prepares the uterus for pregnancy (progestos) — hence pro-gest-erone (-one indicates the kind of chemical substance).

Progesterone is the second main female sex hormone. It has many actions, but the chief ones are that it relaxes smooth (involuntary) muscles; increases the production of the waxy secretions of the skin; and raises the temperature of the body. This is why it is normal for women in the second half of the menstrual cycle to have a temperature of up to 37.4°C (99.5°F). The part of the menstrual cycle after ovulation is called the luteal or the progestational phase. The most important progestational effect of progesterone is its action on the uterus. Progesterone thickens the lining of the uterus, and induces the glands to secrete a nutritious fluid and become succulent, so that a fertilized egg may be nourished during the time it needs to implant in the lining of the womb.

If the egg has not been fertilized and has not implanted into the endometrium, the yellow body in the ovary dies (as do the other stimulated follicles). When this happens, the level of oestrogen and progesterone in the blood falls. This has two effects: firstly, the restraint on the release of gonadotrophin releasing hormone by the hypothalamus is removed, and FSH production by the pituitary gland increases. Secondly, without the stimulation of oestrogen and progesterone, the now thick, juicy lining of the uterus begins to shrink and in doing so, kinks the tiny blood vessels that supply it. The kinked blood vessels (really blood capillaries) break, and patchy bleeding occurs in the deeper layers of the lining. This separates the lining above the blood; it crumbles and is shed into the uterine cavity, together with blood. Within a few hours, the amount of menstrual discharge in the uterine cavity is such that the uterus contracts, expelling it through the cervix into the vagina. Menstruation has begun.

Menstruation is the only visible demonstration of the hormonal relationships that occur in a woman's body each month. These relationships are important; if they are altered menstruation may become less or more frequent, heavier or lighter, last for longer or shorter periods and be painful or painless.

## HORMONAL CHANGES BEFORE AND AFTER THE MENOPAUSE

From the age of about 40, the precise interaction between the various hormones that 'control' menstruation begin to alter for reasons that are not yet understood. The most likely explanation is that the cells surrounding the follicles in the ovaries begin to become less receptive to the circulating pituitary hormones. In an effort to overcome the poor response, increasing amounts of FSH begin to be secreted, and the relative proportion of FSH and LH alters. This in turn leads to less frequent ovulation and, in some women, menstruation becomes irregular. As the years pass, the egg cells in the ovaries begin to disappear and their response to FSH is further reduced. In an attempt to stimulate the egg cells to grow, more FSH is secreted and its level in the blood rises, while a little later the level of LH also rises. Eventually, either all the egg cells disappear or most become unresponsive to the pituitary hormones, and the level of oestrogen secreted by them falls. The uterus is no longer stimulated and menstruation ceases. The woman has reached her menopause (Fig. 2.6).

From this it follows that the menopause is associated with two major hormone changes. The first is that the level of the pituitary hormones FSH and LH becomes higher and the second is that the level of oestrogen becomes lower than during the reproductive years. Many of the symptoms of the menopause appear to be related to these hormonal changes.

Although the general trend of the hormonal changes is for the levels of the pituitary hormones to rise and the oestrogen levels to fall, very wide variations occur from day to day in the same woman and between women in their 40s. This means that measuring the levels of the hormones in the blood may not be helpful in determining that the menopause has been reached. Moreover, if menopausal symptoms occur, treatment often relieves them, irrespective of the hormone levels.

After the menopause the levels of FSH and LH increase considerably (Fig. 2.7), while that of oestrogen falls. Oestrogen continues to be produced in varying amounts by postmenopausal women. The ovaries no longer produce oestrogen but continue to secrete

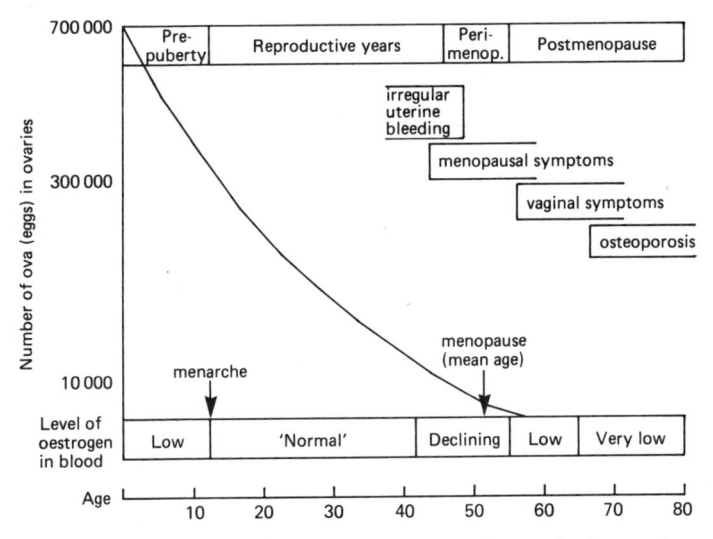

Figure 2.6: Relationship between number of eggs in the ovaries, oestrogen levels in blood and perimenopausal and postmenopausal symptoms

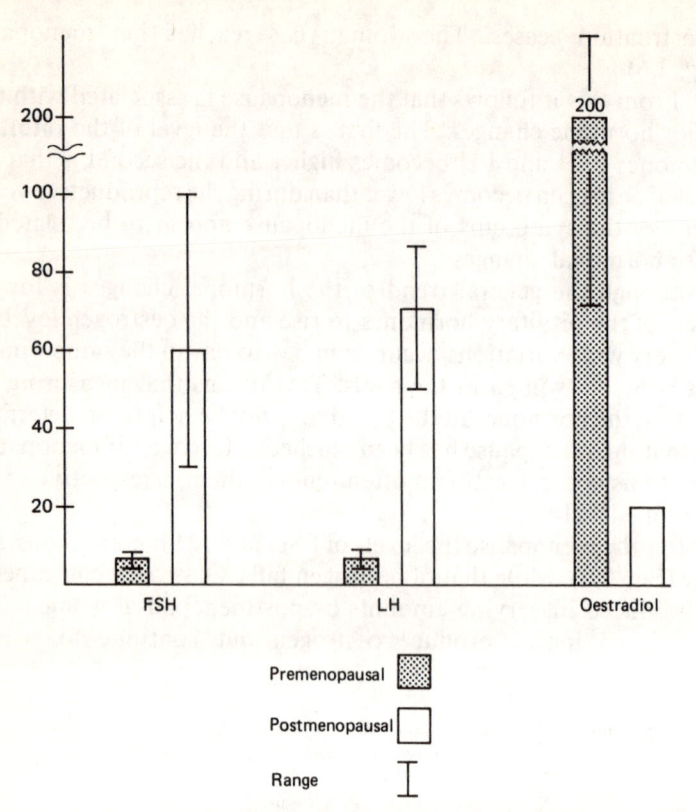

Figure 2.7: Levels of hormones in the blood in the years before and after menopause

substances from which oestrogen is made, as does one other organ in the body, the adrenal gland. These substances are converted into oestrogen in the fat that insulates the body. The more fat that covers a woman's body, the greater is the degree of conversion. The ovaries also produce the male hormone testosterone, as does the adrenal gland. The level of testosterone in the blood falls slightly after the menopause, but relative to the quantity of oestrogen rises somewhat. This may be a reason for the increased facial hair that occurs in some postmenopausal women.

# 3

# A WOMAN IN HER FORTIES

Apart from the relationship problems a woman may have with her husband or partner and with her children, as she strives to find her own identity as an individual rather than a mother, a help mate, a carer and a support for her husband or partner, three other women's health issues may occur.

These are:
   (i) how to avoid a further pregnancy,
   (ii) the continuing distress caused by the premenstrual syndrome (premenstrual tension), and
   (iii) the problem of menstrual changes due to the fluctuating sex hormones which occur during this period of a woman's life.

## FERTILITY AND CONTRACEPTION AFTER 40

After the age of 40, a woman's capacity to procreate (called her fecundity) declines. It might be thought that the main reason for this decline in fecundity is that the frequency of sexual intercourse of many couples drops by 50 per cent between the ages of 20 and 40, particularly if they have had a long-lasting relationship. This is not the main reason for the decline in fecundity.

Studies of women having artificial insemination using a donor's semen, and women in IVF programmes, show that women over the age of 36, and particularly over the age of 40, are less likely than younger women to conceive following these procedures. Either the woman's ova (being of poorer quality as they age), are less able to be fertilized by the sperm or the very early development of the embryo fails to progress.

In spite of the decline in fertility, over 50 per cent of women over the age of 40, who wish to conceive, become pregnant. If they conceive, they face additional hazards, although with good antenatal supervision, their impact is reduced. Women over the age of 40 are more likely than younger women to miscarry; they are more likely to develop a high blood pressure; they are more likely to develop 'pregnancy diabetes.' Their babies have a higher chance of having Downs syndrome (1 in 40, compared with 1 in 1200, if the woman is aged less than 30).

None of these problems is insurmountable. Downs syndrome can be detected early in pregnancy, and if the couple wish, the pregnancy can be terminated. Good antenatal care will detect a rise in blood pressure sufficiently early for treatment to be given, and women over 40 are 'screened' for pregnancy diabetes, which, if found, is controlled.

Nevertheless, statistics show that most women have completed their family by the age of 35 and have been using one or other of the available methods of contraception since that time. Studies in Britain have shown that women choose different contraceptive methods as they grow older (Fig. 3.1).

In their twenties, most women choose to use the Pill or their partner uses a condom. By the age of 40, most women or their partners have chosen to have a permanent method of birth control, either a tubal ligation or a vasectomy. Fewer than 20 per cent of the couples choose condoms or the Pill.

Women after the age of 40, who menstruate regularly, should be aware that they may still be ovulating and at risk of pregnancy — as are some women in their 40s who think that they have reached the menopause — but suddenly have unexpected, unpredictable episodes of menstrual bleeding. These women may find that the Pill, which regulates menstruation as well as protecting against pregnancy, is the preferred contraceptive method.

## The Pill

About 15 years ago, a report from the Royal College of General Practitioners Oral Contraceptive Study, suggested that women over the age of 35 who continued to take the oral contraceptives then available, were at increased risk of dying from cardiovascular disease, particularly clots in the veins which are carried to the lungs (thromboembolism). The reason was that the Pill altered some of the blood-clotting factors to make the blood more likely to clot. The publicity engendered by this report was immense.

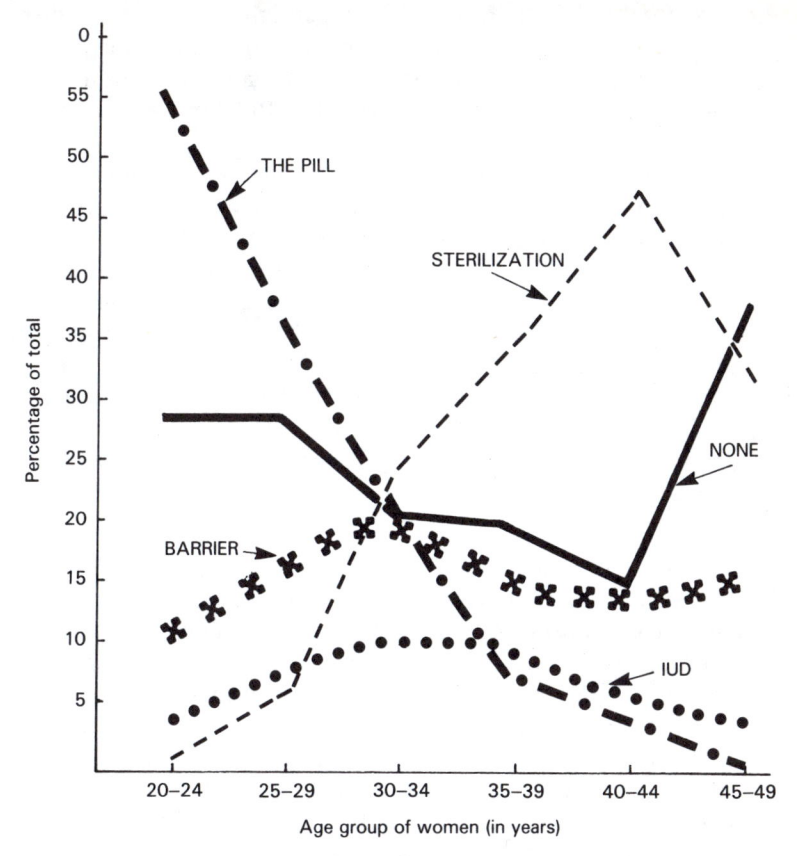

Figure 3.1:

The reason appeared to be that one of the components of the Pill, oestrogen, was implicated in the increased risk of thromboembolism, whilst progestogen, the other component of the Pill, was believed to be the reason for the slightly increased risk of a heart attack. Later studies showed that smoking was an even more important risk factor for both conditions.

Since that day, new oral contraceptives have been developed in which the dose of oestrogen is lower, and new progestogens are used which do not increase the risk of heart attacks.

The current view is that if a woman is not a smoker and is not obese, she can quite safely continue taking one of the new low-dose

Pills (preferably in which the progestogen is either desogestrel or gestodene), up to the menopause. But as the Pill alters the blood-clotting factors, it is recommended that a woman who needs to have a major operation should stop taking the Pill four weeks before surgery, if this is possible.

It may be asked, why stop at the menopause? In fact, some authorities continue with the Pill after that time to control the symptoms of the menopausal years. Most physicians suggest that the woman changes from the Pill, which contains an oestrogen which lingers a long time in the liver, and chooses a more 'natural' oestrogen which is metabolized more naturally in the liver. The reverse of this statement may be asked. Why not give a Pill containing a natural oestrogen in place of the existing Pills? The answer is that the menopausal hormone treatments, in the doses used, are not sufficient to suppress ovulation and prevent pregnancy consistently, and are more expensive.

### The Condom and Diaphragm

Some couples may prefer to avoid any possible risk, however small, of using an oral contraceptive. For them, the barrier methods may be appropriate. Many men do not like using a condom claiming that it is tight fitting, and reduces sensation during sexual intercourse. A new loose-fitting condom has been developed which may be found more satisfactory when it becomes generally available.

The woman may chose to use a diaphragm, or a new device which has been called a female condom, although research shows that most women do not want to use this device.

## THE PREMENSTRUAL SYNDROME

Most women know that they feel more irritable, angry or depressed and may have uncomfortable breasts or a bloated abdomen during the week before menstruation. In a few women, these mood or physical symptoms are severe, and disrupt the woman's life or put a strain on her relationships, particularly with her husband or partner or with her children. During menstruation, the symptoms disappear and the woman is free of them for a week or 10 days. A woman who has this pattern of symptoms has the premenstrual syndrome or PMS. Using these strict criteria, between 5 and 10 per cent of women aged 20 to 45 have been found to have PMS.

The mood and physical symptoms begin in the 2 weeks before menstruation and disappear during menstruation. As just mentioned, in the first week after menstruation they are no longer present and many women feel a sense of euphoria — the so-called 'post menstrual syndrome'.

The onset of PMS may follow the birth of a child or a life crisis, but most women are unable to identify a trigger. PMS becomes a problem to most women when they are in their late 20s or their 30s but it continues, and often gets worse, in a woman's early 40s.

We have found in our studies of PMS that most women put up with PMS or try 'over-the-counter' remedies for about 5 years before seeking professional help.

The mood changes are many. Women with PMS may say that they feel irritable, fidgety, indecisive, confused, disappointed, easily upset (with inexplicable bouts of crying), aggressive or pessimistic. Some women have swings in mood with episodes of irrational anger or depression. Other women become dissatisfied about their appearance or lose any sexual desire during this time.

The physical changes are as varied as the mood changes, the main ones reported being: breast discomfort with tenderness or pain; abdominal bloating with tenderness or pain; dizziness; and increased or decreased appetite.

Our research showed that the mood changes could be placed in a single group: 'general negative mood'; and the physical symptoms could be put into two clusters. The first cluster started soon after ovulation and included breast symptoms, abdominal fullness and an increased appetite. The second cluster of symptoms, which included headache, fatigue, abdominal discomfort or pain and menstrual cramps started a few days before menstruation and peaked during menstruation. We have given this symptom cluster the name 'perimenstrual syndrome'. PMS may merge with the perimenstrual syndrome, or the perimenstrual syndrome may be discrete. If it is discrete, antiprostaglandin treatment often helps, the woman taking the chosen anti prostaglandin as soon as the symptoms start, one or two days before menstruation.

Our research showed that many women who had PMS found it helpful if the woman kept a daily diary of symptoms for 3 menstrual cycles (Fig. 3.3). This diary enabled women to differentiate between their various groups of symptoms and, when it was reviewed by the woman and her health advisor, gave insight into the problems, which could then be discussed. We also found that by keeping the

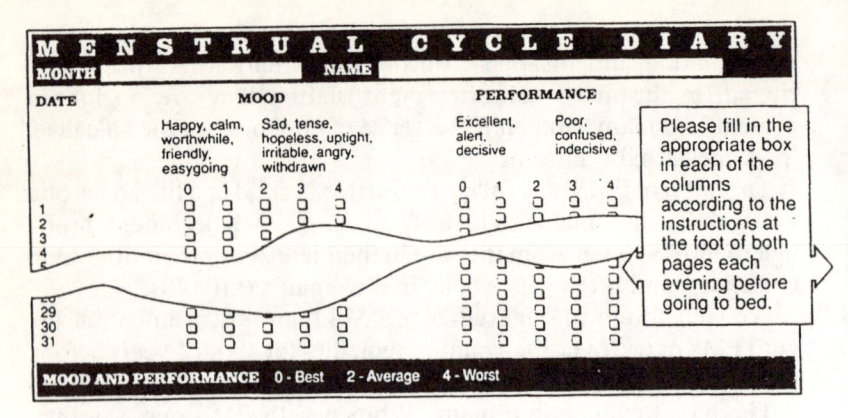

Figure 3.2: Menstrual cycle diary to be completed by the patient over 3 consecutive months

diary many women found that the severity of PMS varied from month to month, and often decreased as the woman became more aware of the problems.

The first medical report of PMS (then called PMT), appeared in the medical literature in 1931, although there can be no doubt that many women had the symptoms long before that time. In the past 60 years, much research and investigation has been made to find the cause of PMS, but in spite of some so-called 'break throughs', its cause is not known.

PMS is a psychosomatic condition, namely a condition in which the mind influences the body and the body influences the mind. The

Table 3.1: Treatments for PMS which are effective for some women who have PMS

| | | |
|---|---|---|
| 1 | Oral contraceptives | Some women report being helped but others say that the PMS is worse. |
| 2 | Progesterone given vaginally | Anecdotally found helpful, but scientific studies found it no better than placebo |
| 3 | Progestogens | Scientific studies shown to be of no benefit |
| 4 | Danazol, a drug which supresses ovarian function | Appears effective, but has side effects (greasy skin, acne, weight gain) which many women find unacceptable |
| 5 | Bromocriptine (Parlodel) | Helps severe breast symptoms but may cause headaches, dizziness and nausea |
| 6 | Vitamin $B_6$ (pyridoxine) | An over-the-counter treatment. Helps some women. Should not be taken in a dose of more than 100 mg a day as may cause nerve damage |
| 7 | Evening primrose oil | An over-the-counter drug, popular but no scientific proof of its value |
| 8 | Spironolactone (a diuretic) | May be of help but doubtful benefits in scientific studies |
| 9 | Antiprostaglandins (Ponstan, Naprogesic Voltarin) | Of value in treating perimenstrual physical symptoms, (See Cluster 2, page 23). |

most likely cause of the interactions is that in some women, the fluctuating levels of oestrogen produced by the woman's ovaries lead to changes in brain chemistry, particularly the release in the brain of substances called endorphins. But at this time, this is speculative.

It is known that women do not have PMS when they are pregnant and when they reach the menopause, which suggests that *fluctuating* oestrogen levels in the body may be a factor. The theory obtained stronger support from two studies made in Canada. Thirty-six women who had incapacitating PMS, which had failed to respond to all available treatments, chose to have a hysterectomy and removal of their ovaries. Because it was realized that the women would get severe menopausal symptoms after surgery, each woman was given an oestrogen implant (see page 76). The implant releases oestrogen slowly into the tissues and blood so that a constant blood level is obtained. The results were most satisfying to each woman: she no longer had severe, incapacitating PMS.

It would be ridiculous to suggest that all women with severe PMS should have their ovaries removed, and for other women a variety of treatments have been suggested (Table 3.1). These treatments work for some women, but so does a placebo, that is, a pill containing a chemically inert substance such as sugar, which the patient thinks will help relieve symptoms. It is unfortunate that the treatments have rarely been subjected to scientific clinical investigation, so the beneficial results reported by enthusiasts tend to be exaggerated.

The theory that fluctuating levels of oestrogen may be a reason for PMS has led to experiments in which an oestrogen implant is injected beneath the skin of a woman's abdomen. As this quantity of oestrogen may stimulate the endometrium (the uterine lining), and perhaps cause cancer, the woman has to take a progestogen tablet (see page 69) for 12 days each month. This causes a 'menstruation' in which the endometrial cells are shed and discharged, and new cells grow in the next menstrual cycle.

Another study in progress is to suppress ovulation, and to maintain a steady level of oestrogen by using a transdermal system, or patch. This is a recognised treatment for menopausal symptoms and is discussed on page 74. If the woman has not had a hysterectomy, she also requires to take progestogen tablets for 12 days a month to induce 'menstruation'.

The results of these studies are awaited to see if these treatments offer a cure for PMS. However, as PMS is a psychosomatic condition, the involvement of the woman in the management of the PMS is essential. Women with severe PMS are helped if they keep the diary, and obtain information and counselling from a health professional or a support group.

Relaxation techniques (one is described on page 62), and exercise programmes help. Drugs should be avoided until these methods have been tried.

## MENSTRUAL DISTURBANCES IN THE FORTIES

In the years before the menopause, many women respond to the fluctuating but declining circulating levels of oestrogen by developing menstrual disturbances. The length of the menstrual cycle may change, becoming longer or shorter — in other words, the interval between the start of one menstrual period and the next becomes longer or shorter. In other women, menstruation may occur at unpredictable intervals.

These changes affect about two-thirds of women to a greater or lesser degree, and only one-third of women have regular periods which suddenly cease, never to return.

As well as changes in the length of the menstrual cycle, many women in their 40s may observe a change in the amount and duration of menstrual flow. If the flow diminishes most women are generally relieved, but if it becomes excessive, with clots and cramps, the woman may be considerably discommoded.

If the periods become less frequent, because of the lower blood level of oestrogen, a loss of bone (see page 106) may occur. Some doctors now recommend that the woman whose menstrual periods are becoming less frequent or are irregular, either takes one of the low-dose pills or is started on hormone replacement treatment or HRT. Hormone replacement treatment does not increase the risk of a clot in a vein (as sometimes occurs if the woman takes the Pill, particularly if she smokes), but, as mentioned earlier, the dose of oestrogen in HRT may be insufficient to protect her against a pregnancy. If she chooses HRT, she or her partner should use another contraceptive method as well.

If the menstrual periods becomes heavy or irregular, a woman in her forties would be wise to visit a doctor.

Some women who have heavy periods are found to have muscular enlargements of the uterus, called myomata or fibroids; very few will be found to have a uterine cancer. These two conditions generally require surgery — hysterectomy being favoured.

Most women who have heavy menstrual periods (menorrhagia), do not have large fibroids or uterine cancer and various treatments are available from which the woman should have the opportunity to choose.

In most cases, the doctor will suggest that a 'diagnostic curettage' is made, and may also suggest that an ultrasound picture of the pelvic organs is taken. The curettage is made so that most of the endometrium may be removed from the uterus and sent for examination by a pathologist. The pathologist is able to exclude endometrial cancer and to describe any abnormality in the endometrium so that appropriate treatment can be given. Curettage needs admission to hospital and a general anaesthetic.

The ultrasound picture is made by introducing a small plastic object (about the size of a sausage) into the woman's vagina. This is connected to the ultrasound machine and the picture of the genital organs is displayed instantly. If there is a fibroid, it will be visible and the thickness of the endometrium can be measured to try and determine if a cancer is present. The procedure is painless.

These procedures are being replaced increasingly by hysteroscopy and endometrial biospy. A hysteroscope is a very narrow telescope (about the size of a medium knitting needle) which is introduced into a woman's uterus through her cervix. As the instrument is so narrow it rarely causes pain. Once the hysteroscope is in the uterus, the doctor can inspect its cavity and take samples of any areas which are suspicious. Hysteroscopy is made in the doctor's rooms or clinic, and the woman neither requires admission to hospital nor a general anaesthetic.

Treatment of the heavy uterine bleeding depends on the findings. In most cases, a fibroid requires hysterectomy, but if small fibroids are present, they may be treated by removing them from the uterus. Endometrial cancer requires hysterectomy.

As mentioned previously, most women in their 40s have neither of these conditions and the problem is one of heavy menstrual bleeding from a normal uterus, which is called 'dysfunctional uterine bleeding'.

The woman has several options for treating dysfunctional uterine bleeding. After discussion with her doctor, she may choose:

(i) to use hormones which are often successful in curing the condition.
(ii) to have a hysterectomy; or
(iii) to have a new procedure called endometrial ablation.

These options will now be considered.

Hormone Treatment

The first treatment which a woman may choose, is to control her menstrual problem using hormones. If this is her choice, a progestogen is usually given, and the woman takes tablets of norethisterone (Primolut–N), or medroxyprogesterone (Provera), from day 5 to day 25 of her menstrual cycle for at least 6 months. She may expect a light bleed each month within 5 days of stopping the tablets.

If the heavy menstrual periods are not relieved, different hormonal regimens may be tried. Two of these treatments are for the woman to take one of the new progestogens, gestrinone, twice a week, for 3 to 6 months, or a drug called danazol, which is taken three times a day for 3 months. These treatments generally lead to amenorrhoea after the first or second month.

## Hysterectomy

The woman may choose to have a hysterectomy. At this age, her ovaries need not be removed, unless they are diseased, so that most women will not suffer from severe, sudden menopausal symptoms. Unfortunately, the ovaries of about a quarter of women who are aged 45 or younger when they have the operation cease to function within 3 years, with the result that the woman may reach the menopause prematurely. This may be a result of the operation, if the blood supply of the ovaries was reduced by the surgery, but in other cases, no reason has been found. Provided that the woman seeks treatment and is given oestrogen replacement, the symptoms of the menopause are relieved satisfactorily.

Hysterectomy is one of the most common operations made on women. In the USA, it has been estimated that over 60 per cent of women will have had a hysterectomy by the age of 70. In the UK, over 40 000 hysterectomies are performed each year. Hysterectomy is a safe operation today, fewer than 6 women in every 10 000 having the operation die. After the operation a few women develop wound infection, and some have problems of urination, either having to pass urine more frequently, or having to respond quickly when they get the urge to pass urine. These urinary problems may persist for some months.

Hysterectomy may be followed by a psychological problem, the woman becoming anxious that she has been mutilated sexually, is less feminine, and will grow old quickly. This may be the reason that only one third of French women have a hysterectomy compared with American women. It is also interesting to note that 60 per cent of the American women who have a hysterectomy are under the age of 44. A reason for the difference in the rate of hysterectomy between the USA and France is that American surgeons tend to view medicine as a battle, in which the doctor has to fight to relieve the person, and in which early intervention is preferable to waiting, as results need to be obtained quickly. French doctors, on the other hand, prefer waiting, and using 'gentle therapies' — at least initially. British and Australian doctors have attitudes somewhere between the American and French doctors.

The feeling of mutilation is reduced or eliminated if, before the operation, the woman has been given some pamphlets or a book to read and then has had the opportunity to talk with the doctor or a counsellor about her feelings and fears, and to discuss the hysterectomy with him or her.

Several myths persist about what happens to a woman after a hysterectomy. The first myth is that after hysterectomy, a woman will not enjoy sex as much, that her sexual desire decreases, that intercourse will be painful or that the woman will not reach orgasm as frequently as before. In most cases these symptoms are not due to the surgery, but the woman may find help if she talks to a counsellor. One reason for the complaints is that the woman may not be certain about her anatomy, and may believe that the removal of her uterus may shorten or narrow her vagina, so that she expects intercourse to be painful. In fact, the vagina is increased in length slightly following hysterectomy. It is true that the cervix is removed, but the contribution of the secretions of the cervix to vaginal lubrication is small, and the movement of the cervix by the man's penis thrusting, is only a minor factor in producing an orgasm.

The second myth is that following hysterectomy a woman becomes depressed. This is untrue. Only two groups of women are more likely to be depressed after hysterectomy. These are women who have been depressed before hysterectomy, and a few women who did not have the opportunity to discuss with their doctor the reasons for the hysterectomy and possible alternative treatments before the operation was performed.

A third myth is that a hysterectomy makes a woman fat. Obesity only occurs after hysterectomy if the woman overeats and takes no exercise.

Most women are well satisfied by the results of hysterectomy, but some are not. Therefore, it is important for a woman to be told of the alternatives to hysterectomy, which are now available.

Endometrial removal (ablation)
There are alternatives to hysterectomy, which may be suggested by a doctor if a woman complains of heavy or irregular menstruation. These alternative procedures are less invasive and recovery from them is quicker.

The procedures involve destroying (ablating), the endometrium using a laser, or an instrument called a resectoscope which uses an electrically heated diathermy loop or a roller ball (often used without hysteroscopic vision), to destroy the endometrium.

The operations are performed by introducing a hysteroscope (a small telescope) into the uterus through the cervix. The hysteroscope enables the gynaecologist to visualize the entire endometrium (often by video monitoring), and then resect it or laser it under vision, which makes the operation safe. The patient may choose to have a general anaesthetic or may be sedated, and the operation performed under local anaesthesia. The woman can leave hospital when she feels ready to do so, many choosing to go home the same day, although some prefer to stay in hospital for one or two days.

Most gynaecologists treat the woman with danazol 200 mg three times a day for 4 to 6 weeks before the operation. This drug reduces the thickness of the endometrium and makes the operation easier.

The technique is new, but if the gynaecologist is experienced, early results show that over half of women evaluated 1 year after the procedure cease to have periods following it, 30 per cent have light periods and 15 per cent are not helped. These women may choose to have a repeat of the endometrial ablation or a hysterectomy.

Over three quarters of women say that they are pleased with the result. A study which followed women for 2 years after the treatment found that menstrual problems had improved in 90 per cent of the women, and one woman in three had ceased to have menstrual periods.

It has to be said that treatments which remove the endometrium are still experimental, as there is no information at present about the long-term efficacy, or of possible complications of any of them. If they prove ineffective, the woman may then choose to have a hysterectomy.

Other innovative treatments are being studied. For example, a hormone releasing intrauterine device is under investigation. The IUD is inserted into the uterus and releases a small amount of a progestogen each day for 5 years. Early studies show that most women cease to have heavy periods within 2 months of having the IUD placed in the uterus. The IUD continues to release tiny quantities of progestogen for 5 years, and protects the woman against pregnancy, as well as solving her menstrual problem.

These techniques give a woman more choices in making a decision, and with the help of her doctor, how she would like to have her complaint of menstrual disturbance treated.

# 4
# HEALTHY EATING IN THE MIDDLE YEARS

As people grow older there is a tendency for them to put on weight, women being more affected than men. Studies in the USA show that an average white woman gains 10 kg between the ages of 15 and 50 (Fig. 4.1). By the age of the menopause, about 30 per cent of women are overweight and about 20 per cent are obese. Obesity carries certain health hazards, such as an increased chance of developing mature-onset diabetes; an increased chance of developing gall bladder disease; a greater likelihood of developing high blood pressure, and a greater chance of having a heart attack or a stroke. Obesity also means that if a woman develops arthritis, the strain on the affected joint is increased and the disability is greater.

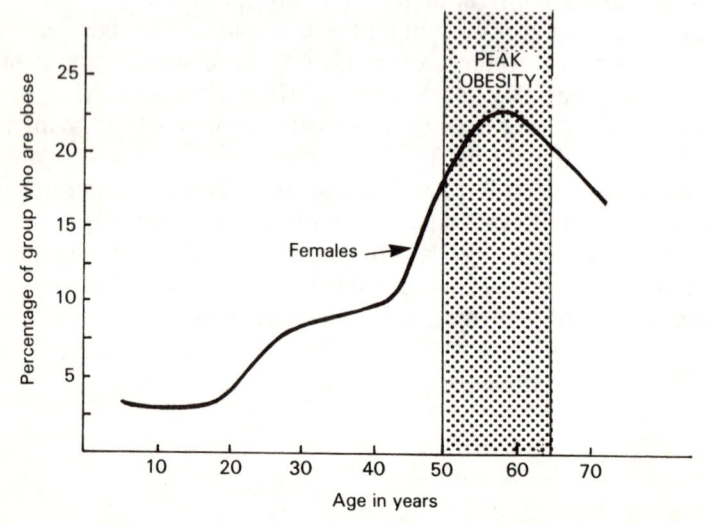

Figure 4.1: Increasing obesity with increasing age

Women are prone to put on weight in middle age for three main reasons. First, they are likely to be less active than when younger. Second, as a woman grows older, her metabolism becomes more efficient. This means that she uses less energy to undertake an activity than she did when she was in her twenties. Third, women are more likely than men to indulge in sweetened drinks (including coffee and tea) and to eat energy-rich snacks between meals.

The contribution of a balanced diet to health is being increasingly recognized, and each year an expert committee in some developed country issues a report suggesting the most appropriate mix of food that should be eaten for health. Unfortunately, the advice is often too obscure to be followed, or makes eating too unpalatable, so the recommendations are largely ignored by people in the community.

## DIETARY PRINCIPLES

It is important for a woman passing through the menopause, as in other periods of her life, to eat a healthy diet. It is known that only 10 per cent of obese people who decide to diet are able to reduce their weight by more than 10 kg (22 lbs), and fewer are able to maintain the lower weight for a year or longer. The reason is that many diets are dull, or 'faddish', or inappropriate. For this reason, rather than prescribe a diet, the principles of a healthy, balanced diet will be given in this chapter, and the reader may then choose whether or not to follow these principles.

If you want to eat a healthy diet (see Fig. 4.2), you should try to follow these recommendations:

- Limit the amount of fat in your diet by choosing lean meat, usually by grilling food rather than frying it, and by limiting the quantity of cakes and biscuits that you eat.
- Reduce the amount of sugar you eat, including sugar 'hidden' in cakes, confectionery and soft drinks.
- Eat more 'complex' carbohydrates, that is eat more wholegrain bread, more oatmeal, more vegetables and more fruit. This increases the amount of fibre in your diet (and is preferable to adding wheat bran to your diet).
- Use less salt by reducing the amount used in cooking and by trying not to add salt to the food on your plate.
- Increase your intake of calcium.

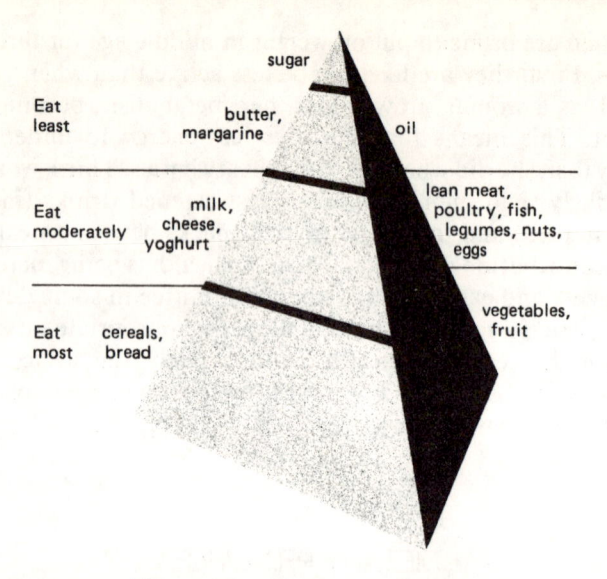

Figure 4.2: Healthy diet pyramid

## Reducing dietary fat

In Australia and Britain, about 38 per cent of the total energy eaten comes from fat. Nutritionists recommend that the percentage should be reduced to 34 per cent. Fat carries twice as much energy as carbohydrates and this is stored in the body, so that the person may become obese. Also, fats, particularly saturated fats, are implicated in the development of heart disease, which becomes more likely to occur as women become postmenopausal. Fat is eaten when you choose fatty meat, and particularly when you eat fried foods. Fat is also 'hidden' in cakes, shortenings, ice-cream, pastries and biscuits (cookies), and chocolates.

You can reduce the amount of fat you eat, and particularly the amount of the more dangerous saturated fats, relatively easily. And it need not disturb your usual eating habits too much. To do this, you may choose lean beef and mutton and try to avoid processed meats like sausages, which have a high proportion of saturated fat. You should eat more fish and poultry and try to resist the temptation to eat the skin because it is fatty.

Usually when you cook meat, poultry or fish it should be grilled or casseroled rather than fried. It is better to use sunflower seed oil or safflower seed oil rather than lard, beef dripping or olive oil. Lard and dripping have a lot of saturated fat in them and olive oil has a fair amount.

It is preferable to choose polyunsaturated margarine (make sure the margarine you buy is polyunsaturated) rather than butter. But if you enjoy butter you may eat it if you spread it thinly.

It will also help if you eat fewer cakes and less confectionery, as these foods are 'energy rich' and contain hidden fat and hidden sugar.

## Reducing sugar in the diet

Sugar and other 'refined carbohydrates' (that is cereal from which most of the fibre has been removed) are a readily available source of energy, the excess of which is stored as fat and adds to the risk that you will become obese. You can reduce the amount of sugar you eat if you do the following:

- Start by cutting down the number of spoons of sugar you add to your tea or coffee, and over a few weeks cut out all sugar you add to hot drinks. What you are doing is 'desensitizing' your taste buds' demands for a sweet taste. This is also a problem if you choose a sugar substitute. It provides no energy but it does not stop your taste buds demanding a sweet taste.
- If you eat breakfast cereals don't put sugar on them.
- Avoid eating cakes and sweet biscuits, except on special occasions.
- Cut out ordinary soft drinks, drink low-calorie ones instead. They do contain sweeteners, but the amount of cyclamate or saccharin in them is not going to do you any harm.
- Or better, buy citrus fruit and make your own fruit drink instead. The fructose in the fruit will make it sweet enough and you will not need to add additional sucrose.
- If you drink alcohol, choose the lighter (less sugary) varieties of beer and avoid ginger-ale, bitter lemon and tonic in your brandy or gin. The first is very sweet; the others seem to be bitter but in reality are loaded with hidden sugar.
- Stop eating sweets, chocolates and toffees between meals. If you need to chew something, chew an apple.

But don't be obsessive. If you want to eat a cake or a piece of chocolate or some ice-cream or have a soft drink from time to time — you can!

## The need for fibre in the diet

For a long time, fibre, that is the outer part of many cereals, vegetables and fruits, was considered to be of no nutritional value. Now it is known that the lack of fibre in modern Western diets is a contributor to the increase in the 'diseases of civilization', particularly bowel disease. About 120 years ago, Western people changed from wholemeal to white bread and reduced the amount of vegetables and fruit they ate, replacing them with cakes, pastries and sweets. Following this dietary change, certain bowel diseases have been diagnosed more frequently. Appendicitis has increased in incidence, as has diverticular disease of the bowel (which now affects over 40 per cent of middle-aged people). Bowel cancer is increasing, as are intestinal polyps. Today more people develop haemorrhoids (piles),

Table 4.1: Best sources of dietary fibre

|  | Average serving size | Dietary fibre (g) |
|---|---|---|
| *Bread and cereals:* | | |
| All-bran | 30 g (1 oz) | 7.5 |
| Muesli | 60 g (2 oz) | 4.0 |
| Raw bran | 7 g (2½ level tablespoons) | 3.0 |
| Oatmeal | 30 g (1 oz) raw | 2.0 |
| Wholemeal bread | 30 g (1 oz; 1 slice) | 2.5 |
| White bread | 30 g (1 oz; 1 slice) | 1.0 |
| Wholemeal pasta | 60 g (2 oz) dry weight | 5.5 |
| *Fruit:* | | |
| Orange | 180 g (6 oz; 1 piece) | 3.6 |
| Banana | 180 g (6 oz; 1 piece) | 3.5 |
| Apple | 150 g (5 oz; 1 piece) | 3.0 |
| Dates | 30 g (1 oz) | 2.5 |
| *Other:* | | |
| Baked beans | 100 g (3½ oz) | 5.0–8.5 |
| *Vegetables:* | | |
| Broad beans | 100 g (3½ oz) boiled | 4.2 |
| Peanuts | 30 g (1 oz) | 2.5 |
| Spinach | 100 g (3½ oz) | 6.3 |
| Corn | 100 g (3½ oz) | 4.7 |
| Cabbage | 100 g (3½ oz) | 2.5 |
| Potato | 100 g (3½ oz; 1 medium) | 2.0 |

which affect one person in every four over the age of 50. Varicose veins are also more common, affecting 20 per cent of Western women compared with 4 per cent of African women.

The discomfort induced by the diseases and the frequency of the diseases themselves can be reduced, especially among menopausal and postmenopausal women, if people increase the quantity of fibre in their diet, so that they eat more than 30 g a day.

## Increasing fibre in the diet

Eat more oatmeal (porridge) and wholegrain bread instead of white bread. This is important as fibre from cereals is better utilized than fibre from vegetables or fruit. But so that you eat a varied diet, choose green vegetables or fruit some days. On other days, you may choose to eat root vegetables or, if you like them, baked beans from time to time, as they are rich in fibre (Table 4.1). In other words, you should eat more grain cereal, vegetables and fruit (including the skins of apples and stone fruit) than you have been accustomed to

Table 4.2: Calcium content of typical average servings of common foods

| Food | Calcium (mg) | Serving size |
|---|---|---|
| Milk (whole or skimmed) | 280 | 250 mL |
| Yoghurt | 310 | 200 g |
| Swiss cheese | 285 | 30 g |
| Cheddar cheese | 260 | 30 g |
| Processed cheese | 205 | 30 g |
| Cottage cheese | 190 | 200 g |
| Canned salmon | 110 | ¼ cup |
| Broccoli | 60 | 60 g |
| Orange | 60 | 150 g |
| Fish | 50 | 100 g |
| Baked beans | 40 | 100 g |
| Egg | 30 | 55 g |
| Carrots | 30 | 90 g |
| French beans | 30 | 60 g |
| Bran flakes | 20 | 30 g |
| Steak | 20 | 100 g |
| Bread (slice) | 10 | 25 g |
| Potato | 10 | (large) |

*Source:* Dairy Corporation (NSW).

eat, but less cakes, biscuits, sweets and sugar. If you can, you should eat 120 g (4 oz) or more of green, leafy vegetables or some fresh fruit every day.

## Vitamins and minerals

If you eat a mixed diet, including fresh vegetables and fruit, you will probably obtain all the vitamins you need from your diet. However, you should increase the calcium-containing foods as at menopause calcium is less easily absorbed from the gut and, in consequence, more should be eaten. Lack of calcium is a factor leading to osteoporosis. Foods containing calcium are listed in Table 4.2 and you should make sure that you obtain 1500 mg of calcium a day. If you do not obtain this amount from food, you should take a calcium tablet every evening (see p. 113).

## Avoiding bad food habits

You will feel healthier if you follow the recommendations just made, and if you can avoid the 'bad' food habits listed in Table 4.3.

Table 4.3:   Bad food habits

* Missing meals
* Replacing meals with snacks of poor nutritional quality, such as tea and sweet biscuits
* Constantly nibbling on lollies, sweet biscuits or cakes
* Not using enough milk or cheese
* Eating insufficient meat, fish, chicken or legumes (dried peas, beans, lentils)
* Drinking less than 1 litre (5 cups) of fluid daily
* Replacing meals with alcohol
* Shaking large amounts of salt on food
* Unable to chew because of ill-fitting dentures or poor teeth
* Running out of basic groceries.

## OBESITY IN MIDDLE AGE

As was mentioned on p. 32, when women grow older they tend to put on weight. In the USA, an average white woman gains 10 kg (22 lbs) between the ages of 18 and 50. Surveys in Australia Britain

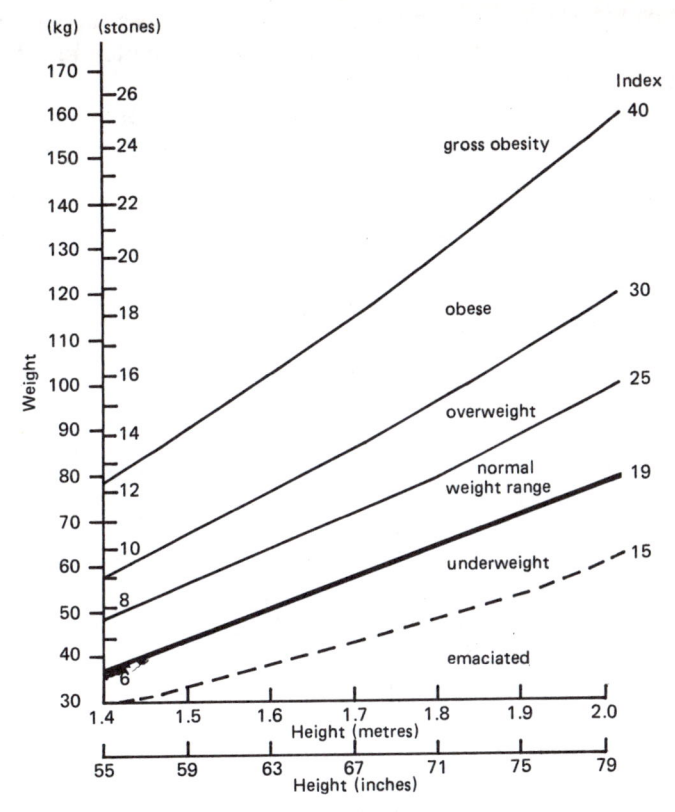

Figure 4.3: The body mass index

and the USA show that by the age of 50, one woman in five is obese. Obesity is defined in several ways. The one that has proved the most accurate and the most useful is the or Body Mass Index (BMI).

This index is calculated by measuring your weight in kilograms and your height in metres. The weight is then divided by the square of the height (Fig. 4.3). This produces a ratio. If your BMI is 30 or more, you are obese. The part of your body in which fat is deposited is important. If you deposit most of the fat on your trunk (your back, abdomen and waist), you are at greater risk of developing heart disease.

Obesity carries health hazards:

- High blood pressure is more common among obese people and if the woman loses weight, her blood pressure is often lowered.
- Stroke is twice as common.
- Heart disease is more common. A woman whose Body Mass Index is 30 or more has twice the risk of developing coronary heart disease compared with a woman whose BMI is in the range 20 to 24.9.
- Diabetes is five times as common and may be cured if the woman loses weight.
- Gall bladder disease is more common and more difficult to treat.
- Osteoarthritis, especially of the hips, knees and back, is more painful if the person is obese.
- Shortness of breath is more common.

For these reasons many menopausal women may wish to lose weight. Losing weight for a short time is relatively easy, but the lost weight is regained rapidly. What an obese person, who is motivated, should try to do is to lose weight slowly and when she reaches the weight she wants, to keep at this weight.

Losing weight permanently is much harder. If it was easy, the annual appearance of new books on 'How to lose weight', or the many magazine articles would not appear!

### A nutritious weight-reducing diet

If you want to lose weight and to maintain your lower weight, you need to change your eating behaviour, so that you eat less permanently but still eat a nutritious diet.

It is easy to read a diet sheet, it is harder to keep to the diet. A diet that is easy to follow and relatively easy to adhere to is given in Table 4.4.

### How to keep to your chosen diet

- Make sure that your diet is palatable and as much like the diet of the rest of your family as you can make it. Unless it is sufficiently varied and tasty, you will become bored with it and will return to your old, familiar eating habits.
- Don't gorge by eating only one large meal a day. You will reduce to, and maintain, a weight in the normal range more easily if you eat several small meals spread through the day.

## Table 4.4: A weight-reducing diet

*Daily allowances of nutrients:*

| | | |
|---|---|---|
| Wholemeal (or enriched bread) | 3 slices | (50 g each) |
| Potatoes (boiled or baked) | 100 g | (3½ oz) |
| *or* Rice (boiled) | 60 g | (2 oz) |
| Milk (skimmed) | 600 ml | (1 pint) |
| Low-fat spread | 12 g | (1½ oz) |

You should eat breakfast (when you may wish to choose from your fruit allowance) and two main meals each day.

Food choices:

*Fruit*  One piece of fruit: apple; orange; half a grapefruit (with sugar); fresh orange juice or orange juice with no added sugar, 100 g; pears; plums; peaches or 100 g of melon. Bananas are NOT allowed.

*Vegetables* (2 portions a day are allowed)
Unlimited amounts: Asparagus; artichoke; beans (green); bean shoots; broccoli; brussel sprouts; cabbage; cauliflower; cucumber; celery; lettuce; mushrooms; mustard and cress; onions; spinach; silver beet

and

50 g of beans (butter, red, haricot); or 50 g of carrots; or of leeks; peas; parsnip; swedes; or turnip.

*Poultry, meat, fish, cheese* (one portion a day) Choose from:

| | | |
|---|---|---|
| | Poultry (remove skin), or game | 60 g |
| *or* | Meat (lean, cut off fat, but still don't fry), minced beef, lean steak, lamb, pork, liver, kidney | 60 g |
| *or* | Fatty fish (salmon, sardines, herrings, trout, mackerel) | 60 g |
| *or* | Cheese (cheddar, camembert, Danish blue, etc.) | 60 g |
| *or* | White fish or shellfish | 60 g |
| *or* | Two eggs | |
| *or* | Cottage cheese | 100 g |

Tea, coffee, water, soda water in unlimited amounts.

*You must avoid:* sugar, sweets, chocolates, jams, honey, pastries and puddings, cakes and buns, ice-cream, canned fruits.

*You should avoid alcoholic drinks*, but if you can't, limit yourself each day to:

| | |
|---|---|
| | Beer 250 ml (10 fluid oz) |
| *or* | Whisky 30 ml (1 fluid oz) |
| *or* | Wine 125 ml (5 fluid oz) |

This diet will provide about 4.2 MJ (1200 kcals) a day and is well balanced in nutrients.

- Don't miss breakfast and don't eat your last meal late at night. The reason for eating several small meals rather than a single, large meal is that smaller meals, eaten at shorter intervals, induce a relatively greater production of body heat, which is then dissipated into the surrounding air. Body heat is produced using energy, and that is what you are trying to do — to use more energy than you ingest.
- Do try to eat your meals at approximately the same time each day. This has the psychological effect of helping you to control your feelings of hunger at times other than meal times.
- Don't raid the fridge between meals.
- Don't keep sweets or bars of chocolate in the house.
- Eat a nutritious diet from a variety of foods in the five food groups.
- Limit your consumption of alcohol. Older people metabolize alcohol less efficiently.

# 5

# THE MENOPAUSE

Menopause means the cessation of menstruation, which occurs because all (or nearly all) the follicles in the ovaries have disappeared and little oestrogen is now being produced. Although menopause has this precise definition, it is commonly used to refer to the years around that event, when the production of the pituitary hormones, FSH and LH and of the sex hormones, oestrogen and progesterone are changing. The more correct term for this period of a woman's life is the 'climacteric', or the perimenopause, but these terms have never 'caught on'. For the purposes of this book, menopause will refer to the cessation of menstruation and to the years around the time.

These years can be as fulfilling to a woman as her earlier years, but in many Western societies, the menopause has been perceived in a singularly negative manner. For example, this quotation is from a book published in France in 1850, and entitled *Hygiene Rules Relative to the Change of Life*.

> Compelled to yield to the power of time, women now cease to exist as the species, and henceforward live only for themselves. Their features are stamped with the impress of age, and their genital organs are sealed with the signet of sterility. The first advice they ought to receive is to reject all sorts of drugs and receipts that are loudly proclaimed by ignorance and puffed by charlatanism. They ought not to sleep upon feather beds, nor in any bed that is too soft and too warm, for such are attended with the disadvantage of exciting the generative organs, which should, henceforth, be left, as far as possible, in a state of inaction.
> It is the dictate of prudence to avoid all such circumstances as might awaken any erotic thoughts in the mind, such as the spectacle of lascivious figures and the reading of passionate novels.

The author of this negative view was, of course, a man! Society's negative view of the menopause and of postmenopausal women may influence the way a woman adjusts to the event.

In the United States, several investigations have been made to find out about women's attitudes towards the menopause. The more recent studies, using a short questionnaire, show that women have a wide range of attitudes towards the menopause. The better educated the woman, the less does she perceive the menopause as a medical condition. Among those women who perceived the menopause as a medical condition and a period when help might be needed, opinion was divided about whether hormone treatment was also needed.

Fewer than 10 per cent of American women believed that the menopause made a woman feel less feminine, or that men saw menopausal women as less desirable.

Several societies in the developing world reward women who reach the menopause. Among certain castes in Rajhastan, women look forward to the menopause with pleasure. With the cessation of menstruation they emerge from Purdah, can move around at will, can talk and joke with men, and acquire a higher status. Similar changes occur for Arabian women, who are restricted to being only with other women in their reproductive years, but can join in social life with men once they have reached the menopause.

Other cultures in Ethiopia, sub-Saharan Africa and Micronesia also respect menopausal women and give them a high social status. Women who live in societies where age is venerated, where grandmothers have a significant role to play in the extended family, where kinship ties are strong, and where menstruation is encompassed with strong prohibitions and taboos, welcome the menopause as a beneficial event, and do not dread it as 'the end of life'.

This does not mean that women in these cultures have no symptoms, which in the West are attributed to the menopause. Studies in several Asian and African countries show that although many women in the menopausal years have symptoms of hot flushes, or vaginal dryness, the symptoms tend to be less severe than those experienced by women living in the developed countries, and most women do not seek help from a doctor. For example, Japanese women associate the menopause (called *konenki*) with growing old, and the actual cessation of menstruation is seen as a relatively minor event in this process. Fewer than 10 per cent complain of hot flushes, but many middle-aged Japanese women complain of headaches, dizziness, shoulder stiffness and other non-specific complaints.

Chinese women do not appear to be concerned about the menopause, most feeling that it is a natural ageing process, and few seek medical help for symptoms. Indonesian women rarely seek help for menopausal complaints, and the complaints reported by women seeking help are usually non-specific.

These findings, from several Asian countries, seem to reflect the situation accurately, but do not provide any information of how the symptoms reported affect the woman's life and her relationship with her husband and family. The effect may be small if the concept of the menopause as a transition towards being elderly may provide psychological and social benefits rather than be disadvantageous. Additional information about the way in which women in the developing nations perceive the menopause could be of great importance to the 350 million women aged 45 or more who live in these countries.

## THE AGE WHEN WOMEN REACH THE MENOPAUSE

In contrast to the onset of menstruation (the menarche), the age of which has declined from about 17 years in the early 19th century to 13 years today, the age of menopause does not seem to have altered over the centuries. In all countries studied, among women of all social classes, whether married or single, childless or having had a large family, half of all women will have ceased to menstruate by the age of 50, and by the age of 56 nearly all women will have reached the menopause. It is normal for some women to reach menopause by the age of 40 or as late as 55 years.

A few women cease to menstruate before the age of 40. These women are described as having a *premature menopause or premature ovarian failure*. Premature menopause occurs because, for some unexplained reason, the eggs remaining in the ovaries disappear and the woman ceases to produce oestrogen. In consequence, she develops the symptoms of the menopause described on page 52, and may also begin to lose bone at a rather rapid rate, which may increase her risk of fractures later in life. These two problems can be corrected if the woman visits a doctor and chooses to start on oestrogen hormone replacement.

Another group of women may reach menopause early. These are women who have had their uterus and ovaries removed because of gynaecological problems. Most gynaecologists try to avoid removing a woman's ovaries if she is under the age of 50, but, in some cases, it is necessary. In others, the doctor leaves the ovaries, but their blood supply is affected by the operation, and the ovaries, cease to produce hormones, prematurely, leading to an *artificial menopause*. Women who have an artificial menopause usually develop more severe menopausal symptoms than women whose menopause occurs naturally, and they are at greater risk of developing osteoporosis.

## WHY HAS THE MENOPAUSE BEEN LARGELY IGNORED BY DOCTORS?

Until 50 years ago, most doctors did not feel it was their responsibility to understand the problems a woman might encounter during the menopausal years. Most doctors perceived menopause as an event through which all women passed, which was not a 'disease', and for which no specific treatment was available. For these reasons menopause could be ignored or treated with sedatives. Such research as was undertaken was neither scientific nor rigorous. In the mid 1930s, with the realization that hormones controlled menstruation and that menopause was in some way due to hormonal changes, doctors became more interested in treating menopausal women, particularly as oestrogen could now be made in the laboratory. In the mid 1940s, oestrogen was selectively prescribed, but a dramatic change now occurred. Two American doctors advanced the opinion that it was every woman's right to be given oestrogen, and that failure to prescribe oestrogen was, in effect, medical negligence. Their argument was based on two doubtful suppositions. The first, as stated by one of the doctors, was that:

> In 1900 the average life expectancy of women in the USA was 48.7 years. Sixty years later this figure has risen to 72.4 years. In other words, in half a century 24 years have been added to a woman's life, but the menopause still occurs at the same time. At the turn of the century Mrs Average launched her family and then died in her 40s, like a spent rocket, whilst today she has another 20 to 30 years of life.

The response to this supposition is as follows: in 1900, the *average* life expectancy at *birth* was low because many females died in childhood or young adulthood. Life expectancy at birth has increased by 24 years or so in the past century. However, if a woman reached the age of 50, her further life expectancy in 1900 was 22 years, while today it is only 6 years more (28 years). In other words, many women in 1900 did live into old age. But many children died from respiratory and gastro-intestinal infections, while young females died from tuberculosis or the effects of childbirth. These illnesses have largely been eliminated in the Western nations, so that many more people avoid the health hazards of childhood and young adulthood to reach menopausal years. Currently, about 50 million women in the USA and Canada are aged 45 or older; in Britain about 9 million, and in Australia and New Zealand about 3 million are in this age group. It can be seen that a considerable number of women will reach the menopause each year and most will live for many years after the menopause. In addition, because of environmental health measures and better medical treatment, the population of older women is growing.

This may be put in another way.

In 17th century Europe, about one woman in three survived childhood, adolescence and the reproductive years to reach menopause. Today, in the developed nations over 90 per cent of women reach menopause, and nearly all of them may expect to live until the age of 65. One in three women reaching 65 will live to celebrate her eightieth birthday. The effect of these factors is that although women reaching the age of 50 today only live on average 6 years longer than women born 100 years ago, there are many more postmenopausal women in the community.

The second argument goes like this:

> Alone of the mammalian species, women live for many years after the end of their reproductive period. During these years they are deprived of the female sex hormones, particularly oestrogen, which leads to a variety of complaints. It is the right of every woman to be prescribed hormonal replacement therapy (HRT) to restore their bodies to health, vigor and beauty.

Although the arguments were not entirely correct, the advice was sound that menopausal women would be wise to consider taking oestrogen for at least ten years and, if they had not had a hysterectomy, a progestogen intermittently. This is because it has been found that although oestrogen does not keep a woman youthful and 'feminine forever', the hormone does relieve the immediate menopausal symptoms and, perhaps more importantly, if taken for a period of years, reduces the risk of heart disease and delays the onset of brittle bones and osteoporosis.

# 6

# PSYCHOLOGICAL CHANGES IN THE MENOPAUSAL YEARS

The years around the menopause are a period of psychological transition. They are years when a woman no longer has menstrual periods each month, or episodes of heavy or irregular bleeding. After the menopause a woman no longer has to bother about contraception to avoid unwanted pregnancies. In a study we made of the attitudes of Australian women to the menopause, positive feelings were expressed by 30 per cent of the women.

Other women see the menopause in a less favourable way. Some women have to adjust to the fact that they can no longer bear a child. Others equate the cessation of menstruation with a loss of femininity, although few women express this view. Some women find the perimenopausal years are difficult because their children have become adults, have left home and have become independent, which the Americans call the 'the empty nest syndrome'. As the children may have moved some distance and are increasingly involved in their own relationships, some women may feel frustrated, angry, or experience anxiety or depression. If this occurs the woman may lose her self-esteem. Other women welcome the autonomy that the departure of the children and the cessation of menstruation provides.

During these years a menopausal woman may have to adjust to marital disharmony. Her husband or partner also may be undergoing a period of transition, as he adjusts to the loss of his dreams and the failure of his youthful ambitions. He may see his future in his job as unstimulating, uninteresting and stretching greyly for a decade or more. He may react to his problem by becoming obsessed with his work, or may become a fitness addict, or resort to alcohol as an escape. He may seek to get rid of his frustrations by 'taking it out' on his wife or by becoming utterly disinterested in her activities. The relationship between the couple may deteriorate so that minor disagreements become major wars. He may react to his confusion and concern about his future by forming a relationship with a younger woman, which tends to confirm his wife's belief that she has become unattractive, which she may blame on her menopause. In these ways the problems of one marriage partner become the problems of the other.

A menopausal woman may have to cope with other problems, which seem to become more serious because of her concern about the menopause. This concern is increased in a society that stresses youth. The woman may believe that the menopause signals 'the end of life' — at least of a life that offered challenges, joys, excitement, as well as dreariness and dissatisfaction.

The feelings of lost hopes, lost femininity, and a general feeling of confusion can be coped with in many ways. Some women cope splendidly on their own, others need a partner's support, often only solving their problems at the expense of the partner. Some women need help from others. Some succumb.

In general, women who have interests outside the home and domesticity cope better than women who only perceive their role in life as that of housewife and mother. Women with more financial, educational, social and cultural resources adjust better because they have more choices in life style at their disposal. In Sweden, at least, the women most affected are housewives with limited education and few interests outside their family. But these findings may not be applicable to women of other nationalities. Women who have a good relationship (including a good sexual relationship) with their partner adjust more easily than women who do not have such a relationship. Sexuality after the menopause is discussed in Chapter 14.

Single women also have problems in the menopausal years. Single women benefit by having a career and social interests, possibly to a greater extent than married women. But often they have no permanent partner to whom they can relate and with whom they can share their concerns. Although a single woman may avoid marital conflict, she may feel that the absence of children leaves her disadvantaged. The menopause is a clear signal to her that she will never have children. Usually a single woman has adapted, some years before she reaches the menopause, to her single status and to the absence of children so that she is no more likely to suffer psychological problems during the menopause than her married sister.

## PSYCHOLOGICAL SYMPTOMS

It will be appreciated from what we have just written that psychological symptoms that occur in the menopausal years are not easy to identify. In addition, as we discuss in Chapter 13, the symptoms are not necessarily *due* to the menopause.

The most common symptoms reported in surveys of menopausal women are: an inability to cope with problems; anxiety; constant (or intermittent) tiredness; irritability and mild depression. But these symptoms are more common in younger and older women (see Chapter 13). In some women the psychological symptoms (at least as judged by recognized anxiety and depression scales) may be aggravated by life stresses. It also appears that the psychological symptoms, particularly anxiety, may exacerbate the physical symptoms such as hot flushes.

## COPING WITH THE PSYCHOLOGICAL CHANGES

The importance of a helpful, supportive, understanding partner in helping a woman through the menopausal years is obvious from the previous discussion. However, in many instances the husband or partner is not equipped to help. A study in Britain in the 1970s showed that at least 25 per cent of the men were unaware of the nature or the extent of their wife's problems. Most of the men had no knowledge of the emotional changes that affect many menopausal women. Many husbands are unaware that a woman needs more love, understanding, encouragement and contact in the menopausal years. Many a husband is unaware that his behaviour may aggravate her emotional upset. The couple should start evaluating their relationship and trying to understand each other better. One way of doing this is to spend more time with each other, doing things that they both enjoy. It is also important that each partner learns to listen to what the other is saying and to talk *with* each other, rather than *at* each other.

Knowledge about the changes that are occurring during the menopausal years also helps the woman to adjust. This knowledge may be obtained from books, but for full effect books need to be supplemented by discussions in 'menopausal groups' or with an informed, empathetic doctor, nurse, clinical psychologist or social worker.

We write about the management of the menopause at greater length in Chapter 8.

# 7

# PHYSICAL SYMPTOMS IN THE MENOPAUSAL YEARS

A problem in identifying which symptoms are due to the reduced levels of the female sex hormone oestrogen and which are due to psychosocial changes is that doctors and psychologists have tended to look at the menopause differently. Doctors, in general, have seen the menopause as a medical condition due to a hormonal deficiency, which should be treated with drugs. Psychologists, on the other hand, have seen the menopause as a period of change, during which a woman has to adapt to and cope with a different role in life.

A few doctors and a few psychologists see menopause as a major transition into old age, or senescence. There is no evidence that the cessation of menstruation and the bodily changes consequent on lowered oestrogen levels is a marker of old age. Menopause is not 'the end of life'; it is only one of many factors demonstrating the ageing process.

However, if women in middle age are to be helped, it would be useful to know how many women have 'disturbing' symptoms during the years around the menopause, and what these symptoms are.

Here some problems arise. It is obvious, if you think about it, that doctors and psychologists who write papers for professional journals or who speak at meetings can only report on the people who have consulted them or have been surveyed by them. This may give other health professionals an unreal picture, as those people who are seen by a doctor or a psychologist may not be representative of the community in which they live, any more than patients who attend a cardiologist are representative of their community, or people visiting a psychologist because of a behavioural problem, of their community. Because of this it is difficult to be sure how many women suffer unpleasant symptoms during the menopausal years. It is also difficult to be sure which of the symptoms are due to the hormonal changes of the menopause and which are coincidental.

## DISTURBING SYMPTOMS DURING THE MENOPAUSE

How many women develop disturbing symptoms in the menopausal years?

In recent years, anecdotal information has been replaced by community studies in an attempt to answer this question.

If the results of the studies are combined, it appears that in the countries of Northern Europe and North America, at least 75 per cent of women suffer some symptoms during the menopause and in one-quarter to one-half the symptoms are associated with physical or emotional discomfort. Of the 75 per cent of women who have symptoms, between one-third and one-half visit a doctor. (Fig. 7.1). The difference in the proportion of women visiting a doctor depends on how women in a particular community perceive the menopause, and on the influence on women of articles about menopause in magazines.

What symptoms are due to the menopause?

This question is harder to answer. This is because symptoms due to menopause may be confused with symptoms due to a change in the woman's life-style or to the ageing process. In past years doctors have tended to list symptoms as diverse as dryness of hair and aching toe-joints as caused by the menopause. However, these doctors were not as undiscriminating as an English doctor who wrote a book in 1870 entitled: *The Change of Life in Health and Disease*. In this book he listed 135 conditions he ascribed to the menopause, ranging from temporary deafness through 'hysterical flatulence' to 'boils in the seat' and 'blind piles'!

Several investigators have tried to obtain more precise information about menopausal symptoms, but unfortunately the way they have done the investigations have made most of the results difficult to interpret. In 1980, an attempt was made to overcome this problem by a group of doctors in Oxfordshire, England. They asked a group of women and men aged 30 to 64 to complete two questionnaires. In all, 1120 women and 510 men were chosen by random sample with about equal numbers in each 5-year age group. The questionnaires were mailed at a 6-week interval asking questions

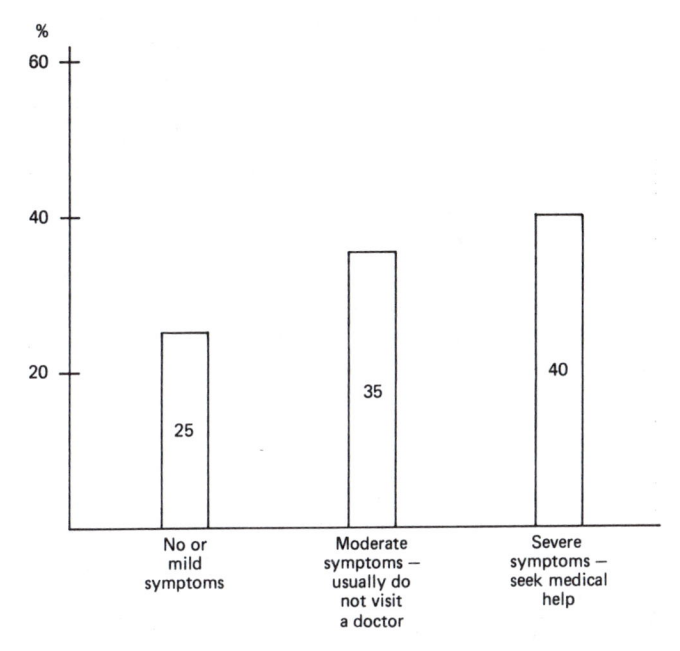

Figure 7.1: Severity of menopausal symptoms

about the person's health. No mention was made that menopausal symptoms were being investigated.

The survey showed that only two sets of symptoms were associated with the menopause. These were hot flushings and night and day sweats. Two years later, two Swedish studies reported similar findings to those from Oxfordshire. The Swedish studies reported one additional group of symptoms associated with the years just after the menopause had been reached. They found that between 15 and 25 per cent of the women they studied complained of vaginal dryness or vaginal 'burning', which in some cases made intercourse painful or impossible. These symptoms only affected a few women in the early postmenopausal years, but the proportion increased as the women became older.

The English doctors found another matter of interest. This was that women aged 45 to 50, who usually had not reached their menopause, complained that they often had difficulty in making decisions and had a greater likelihood of having lost their confidence than younger or older women. These emotional changes might be due to hormonal changes but it is more likely that they are due to a negative cultural perception of menopause. This perception by society and by the woman herself may cause her to lose her belief in her value to herself and to others, and may cause her to lose her self confidence.

The studies from England and Sweden suggest that only two groups of symptoms are caused by the menopause. In the first group are the *vasomotor symptoms* of hot flushes, sweats and insomnia. This sequence often leaves the woman fatigued and forgetful the next day, which are two symptoms often mentioned by menopausal women. The second group includes: *vaginal dryness, discomfort and sometimes burning*. The vaginal symptoms and painful intercourse that occur because of them usually are not severe until 5 or more years after the menopause.

## The vasomotor symptoms

The majority of menopausal women who present to a doctor complain of hot flushes (called hot flashes in the USA). A hot flush has been described by one of our patients as follows:

> At intervals I suddenly get a feeling of heat which starts either in my face and spreads to my neck and upper chest, or begins in my chest and spreads upwards. Occasionally my whole body feels hot. I know it only lasts for a minute or so, but it does disturb me. I keep waiting for the thing to come again. If it happens at night, as it often does, I wake up in a sweat. I throw off the bedclothes and often have to get out of bed and dry myself with a towel, then I can't get back to sleep again. In many of the flushes, I develop red blotches on my neck, and it looks ugly. When the flush finishes, I often feel cold, shiver a bit and feel stupidly weak for a short time. I have begun to hate myself and my flushes. I suppose that this self hate is making me more aware of my body, or something like that, because I now notice that sometimes my heart thumps and thumps and it never did before.

The frequency and severity of hot flushes vary between women. In many women the flushes are mild and infrequent and do not disturb the woman. In others they are so severe they may affect considerably a woman's enjoyment of life and her efficiency at work. Hot flushes precede the actual menopause in about 30 per cent of women (being more common when the periods become irregular) and persist for up to 5 years after menstruation ceases in 20 per cent of women

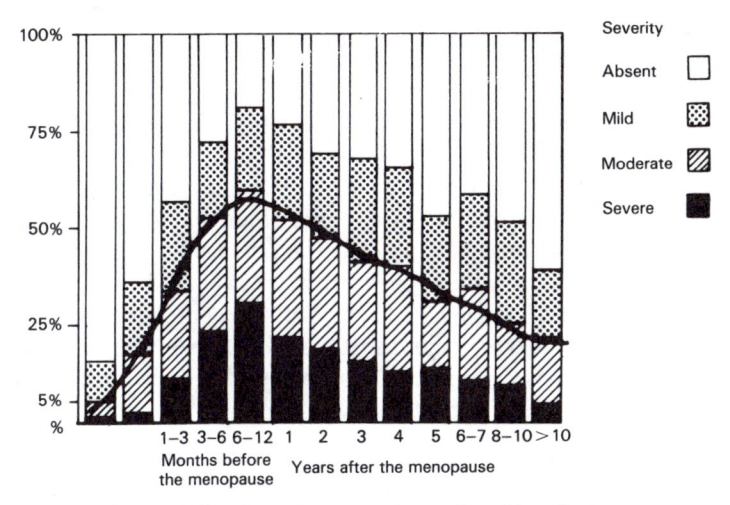

Figure 7.2: Prevalence and severity of hot flushes

(Fig. 7.2). In most women, however, their duration is limited to about one year, starting at the menopause. About 40 per cent of women say that they have no flushes, in 20 per cent they are mild and in 40 per cent they are moderately or severely disturbing to the woman.

What causes hot flushes?

It is known that, following a brief 'warning', there is an increase in blood flow in the tissues beneath the skin and the pulse rate rises, but the blood pressure levels are unaltered. The episode lasts for 2 to 3 minutes, although the blood flow changes persist for longer, during which time sweating may occur. Flushes are associated with low levels of oestrogen but this cannot be the only cause because the flushes usually cease in 2 or 5 years, while the level of oestrogen falls further as the woman grows older. But it is possible that during the transitional period of the early menopause, because of the fall in oestrogen levels in the blood, a woman's vascular system is 'made more sensitive to the effects of certain brain hormones and opium-like substances' so that it is less well controlled. This mechanism would account for the flushes, the sweats, the palpitations and perhaps headache, which some women say is more frequent in the years around the time menstruation ceases.

## The dry painful vagina

One of our patients told us:

> The problem didn't start at my menopause which wasn't really a problem. But a few years later I noticed that my vagina felt dry and on some days I felt a burning feeling inside it. We don't have intercourse often now; my husband is older than me and doesn't seem to want it, but every so often he decides he wants to make love. That isn't really the right word; he's never really made love in recent years. No foreplay, just sex. Well, I accepted that but now I find that when he tries to go inside me it hurts. So I tell him to stop and he gets cranky. He doesn't talk to me for days until he's got over it. I suppose it is part of growing old.

Vaginal dryness, burning, and pain when the woman's husband tries to introduce his penis into her vagina, are symptoms that usually occur for the first time a few years after the menopause, but may occur earlier. Most women do not experience the symptoms, and when present, they vary in severity from woman to woman. They are more common among women who only have intercourse infrequently at long intervals. The cause is a thinning of the vaginal lining and a reduction in the blood flow to the vagina. You may recall that during the reproductive years the vagina is lined by a 'wall' of cells, 30 cells deep. The structure of the vaginal wall depends on oestrogen. After the menopause, with the fall in the level of oestrogen in the blood, the thickness of the vaginal wall decreases, so that it may be 10 cells thick or less. The acidity of the vagina also decreases, allowing more pathogenic bacteria to grow. A reduction in blood flow to the vagina aggravates the problem and the vagina becomes less able to distend. These factors — the reduction in the structures of the vagina and its reduced ability to expand easily — lead to the feeling of dryness and to painful intercourse.

# 8

# HOW TO MANAGE THE MENOPAUSE

The menopause, as well as being a period of hormonal change, is a time of life-change, of renewal, when different aspirations are perceived and different challenges are experienced. For this reason the management of the menopause needs to take into account two interlinked but separate treatments. The first is psychological, the second pharmacological.

The purpose of psychological treatment (talking, psychotherapy or counselling) is to help the woman to understand her body and to become acquainted with the changes it is undergoing as she moves from the reproductive years of her life through the menopausal years into the postmenopausal period.

The purpose of pharmacological treatment is to prescribe hormones and other drugs to treat the menopausal symptoms for which they are specific. Hormone treatment is only appropriate for those symptoms that are related to hormone deficiency, which in most cases is a lack of oestrogen circulating in the woman's body. The two menopausal symptoms likely to respond to oestrogen treatment are the *vasomotor symptoms* of hot flushes, sweats and insomnia; and, usually later in the menopausal years, *vaginal symptoms* of dryness, burning and pain during intercourse. Some doctors and some women believe that oestrogen treatment reduces fatigue and increases sexual desire.

## MANAGEMENT OF THE PSYCHOLOGICAL SYMPTOMS

Many of the symptoms both psychological and physical, experienced by a woman during the menopausal years are relieved if the woman takes into account her general health. During these years a woman may take the opportunity to assess herself and to look at her life-style, so that she can make changes that should result in a more relaxed, healthier and happier life. This approach reduces the impact of many of the symptoms that occur during these years.

Perhaps the most important action a woman can take is to understand what is happening to her body and to know what she may expect. We have found that many women feel that there is insufficient readily available information about the menopause. We also found that women perceived that many health professionals consulted were not particularly helpful, although individual doctors, psychologists or social workers were concerned and helpful.

When consulting a health professional, many women either do not ask about matters that concern them, or the health professional does not raise the issues. For example, women who recently have ceased to menstruate would like to know for how long they should carry a tampon in their handbag in case bleeding suddenly starts. As the menstrual pattern varies so much between individual women, this information is not available. Another question often raised by women is how long the hot flushes will continue, as a woman might be prepared to put up with the inconvenience without hormonal treatment if they only lasted for six months but would not if they persisted for 5 years. The reason that a woman wishes to avoid hormones may be because of the belief that the menopause is a natural event, or because of bad experiences when taking the 'Pill' earlier in life, or anxiety because the media usually only report sensational or adverse findings about hormones. Again, information about the duration of hot flushes in an individual woman is not available. Another matter of concern to many women is when the woman (or her husband or partner) can cease to use contraceptives and be sure that pregnancy will not occur. In our survey, 35 per cent of Australian women worried about pregnancy occurring during the menopausal years.

These examples show the importance for the woman to find a person or a group she feels she can trust and talk with and who will provide her with realistic information and give her the opportunity to discuss the ways in which she thinks she may best be helped.

### Psychological health

Thirty per cent of the women we talked to, in our survey, who had not reached the menopause were apprehensive or anxious about it, while most of the women who had reached the menopause felt that it was 'better' than they had anticipated. In our study, and in a large American community-based study carried out in Massachusetts, over half of the women welcomed the menopause as relief from distressing premenstrual symptoms, from menstruation and from the need to use contraceptive measures to prevent a pregnancy occurring. Another third of the women didn't mind that they had reached the menopause.

Similar findings were made in a survey which has been continuing for the past 10 years in the town of Ede in The Netherlands. In that study, 60 per cent of the women surveyed were pleased that their periods would cease.

Fewer than 15 per cent of the women in the three studies perceived the idea of reaching the menopause as unpleasant, or were sad to have reached the 'change of life'. Most of these women had chosen to see their main role in life as producing, rearing and caring for children. The menopause signalled that this role had largely ceased. The feeling of ceasing to have a significant role after the menopause was increased if the woman's relationship with her partner was unrewarding, and if the woman had few friends and outside interests. It should be stressed that only a very few women had these perceptions.

To many women the menopause also signals that they are getting older. According to women's magazines, getting old is of concern to women as they enter their fourth and fifth decade and particularly their sixth decade. The start of the sixth decade often coincides with menopausal symptoms, and is seen as the major marker of ageing. The menopause does not mean that the woman is old, and that she should now think and behave as an older woman. This was a normal attitude a hundred years ago. It has now largely disappeared, but it persists in some women's minds. If a woman feels that her future stretches out greyly, that she has not done or achieved many of the things she wanted and that her useful life is finished, it often helps if she can talk with other women who have experienced the same problems. Menopause does not signal the end of an active, interesting life or the end of curiosity. It does mark entry into middle age.

Middle age can be a distressing time for some women. A middle-aged woman may realize that she is not as attractive physically as she was when younger; nor is she as physically able to compete with younger women. She may be aware that her relationship with her husband or partner is less than good. The couple may have gone their own ways; they may feel that they have little in common; they no longer talk *with* each other. The woman may no longer even like the man and may wonder how she is going to continue to live with him for the next thirty years or so without a common interest, such as children. She may also wonder how she could manage if she no longer had the financial security he provides. If the woman has no partner the financial problems of middle age may also be present. A single woman may be concerned how to put aside money for retirement or if she is 'made redundant'. She may be concerned about her health, or about the health of a parent for whom she feels responsible.

Children may also be a cause for concern. When a woman reaches the menopausal years, her children are likely to be in their early or mid-twenties, with all the problems that that age can occasion. They may still be involved in risk-taking, of not being responsible, and of being miserable. Whatever advice the woman gives may be seen as wrong, or as interfering, or as not understanding.

Although problems of middle age may occur before, during or after the menopause, many of them can be dealt with by a positive approach.

## A positive approach to the menopause

A woman in the menopausal years is experienced and mature. She has coped with many problems, she has solved many problems, and she can be confident that she can cope in the future. The menopausal years are a period when a woman should consider if it is not time that she stopped playing the self-sacrificing role of always considering her needs last. It is often helpful for a woman to make a list of what she has done for others so far in her life, and what she has done for herself. She may get a considerable surprise! It is a period when a woman should make time to decide what makes her feel good, what is comfortable and what she could do to help herself, both psychologically and physically. It is a period when she should take time to reflect on her priorities. For example, most younger women would list their priorities as baby, toddler, children, husband, housework, job, family life and social life. At the end of the list she puts herself and her needs. Middle age, with the menopause as the trigger, can be a time to reassess her priorities and to make changes. Sometimes it is helpful to make a list of the things the woman would like to do and to make enquiries about how to do them. The list may include hobbies, or further education, or exercise programs, or excursions, or sport.

Having made her decisions, the woman should ensure that she will do the chosen activity even if she has opposition from her husband or family. The menopausal years are a period when a woman may need to become self assertive and relinquish the role of being someone else's prop.

This is not to suggest that she should antagonize her family. It is a time to talk with her husband, or partner, so that they can make changes, if these are needed to make their relationship more enjoyable. The man may have problems too. He may be concerned about his future career, he may be anxious about his retirement, or his health, he may be concerned about the relationship. The menopausal years give the couple the opportunity to look at their lives, to understand each other's problems, and to reassure each other of their love and concern. The opportunity to be self assertive and to give one's own needs a high priority can be stressful. This and the other stresses of middle age can be reduced by talking to an experienced counsellor and by practising a relaxation technique.

Relaxation exercises
The body benefits from active and from passive forms of relaxation. Active relaxation such as exercise and sport (which is not competitive), walking, jogging, gym workouts, dancing, tennis and swimming are all helpful. A woman who decides on active relaxation should chose an activity she enjoys. If it is strenuous activity (such as gym workouts or jogging) she should have a medical check before starting and should build up the activity slowly. Some of the active methods of relaxation benefit the cardiovascular system, others do not. Only those activities that increase the woman's heart rate over a period of 30 minutes are beneficial in this regard. These include brisk walking, jogging, and workouts. Tennis, golf and swimming do not have this effect although they have other benefits, such as stretching muscles and mobilizing joints.

Regular, enjoyable exercise has another positive advantage. There is a tendency for women in their middle years to put on weight. This is because in these years women use energy more effectively. This may seem a paradox but it can be explained. For example, a woman who is 25 may expend so much energy running 100 metres. If she runs the same distance at the same speed in her mid 40s, she will expend less energy, because she utilizes energy more efficiently, and that saved energy is available to be turned into fat. Studies have shown that exercise is nearly as important in losing weight as is prudent eating, which is discussed in Chapter 4.

Regular exercise during the middle years is also thought to reduce the chance that the woman will develop depression (Chapter 13).

Passive relaxation is obtained by 'exercises', which may be done at a community centre or at home. Passive exercises include yoga, meditation, and hypnosis. One form is becoming increasingly popular. This is Tai Chi, which consists of passive relaxation with gentle movements.

A relaxation exercise that is effective in relieving stress and is easy to do is described below.

Relaxation exercise

1 Sit in a comfortable chair or lie down where you are unlikely to be disturbed for a few minutes.
2 Make sure you are comfortable, with your hands and legs uncrossed and with no tight clothing such as shoes or belt.
3 Listen to the sounds around you, for example traffic outside, the clock in the room, the family in another room. If you are aware of these sounds they will not disturb you when you are relaxing.
4 Close your eyes. Although your eyelids may flicker, this will stop soon.
5 Become aware of your breathing.
6 Take a breath and then let the rate of your breathing slow, so it is about the same as when you are asleep. Don't try to force it. Just let it slow down so it is comfortable.
7 Each time you breathe out, let your body relax so you feel limp and floppy and warm and heavy as though you are sinking into the chair or a bed.
8 Keep thinking about your breathing and keep it slowed down.
9 Think of your arm muscles and let them relax. Then think of your leg muscles, then your body muscles, then your neck muscles, your face and forehead muscles — let each group of muscles relax so that you are completely relaxed.
10 Spend no more than 2 minutes doing the exercise, each time you do it.

Try to do this exercise a few times when you do not feel tense. If you find you cannot relax you may wish to join a group that teaches relaxation.

This exercise needs practice — about four to six times a day for a month — so you can use it when you are very tense.

The psychological management of the menopause should take place concurrently with the management of the physical symptoms.

## MANAGEMENT OF THE PHYSICAL SYMPTOMS

Women frequently neglect their own health while ensuring that the health of their children and husband or partner is cared for. The presence of a few menopausal symptoms can provide the opportunity for a woman to look at her own health. If a woman has not seen a doctor for some time, and particularly if she feels run down or easily fatigued, the start of the menopausal symptoms is an ideal time to have a health check-up. The woman should choose a doctor in whom she has confidence and who is willing to spend time to answer her questions, no matter how trivial they may seem. The check-up should include an assessment of the woman's weight and blood pressure, and a Pap smear should be taken if this has not been done in the past year. If a woman has not had a mammogram performed, the value of this painless investigation should be discussed. In middle age a person's sight tends to deteriorate, and referral to an ophthalmologist or an optician may be desirable.

Some menopausal women will benefit by improving their nutrition and their eating habits, and this can be talked about at the time of the check-up. We discuss nutrition in Chapter 4. Women of all ages are concerned about their body shape and body weight. A study made in South Australia found that 40 per cent of middle-aged women had been concerned about their weight and had had problems with weight control since their twenties. Over three-quarters of these women wanted to lose weight from parts of their body, most wanting to lose weight from their stomach, their hips or their thighs. This desire can lead to embarking on a variety of diets, or of deciding to eat only 'healthy foods'. In the South Australian study 43 per cent of the women were dieting at the time of the survey.

During the health check-up the woman may seek advice about her intake of caffeine. Caffeine is a component of coffee and of tea, and is found in other drinks such as chocolate, cocoa and cola drinks, in lesser amounts.

Many women are advised to reduce their intake of caffeine in the menopausal years. The advice is because caffeine may increase irritability, lead to insomnia if taken in the 4 to 6 hours before sleeping, and may be a factor in the development of osteoporosis. These effects probably only arise if the woman drinks excessive amounts of caffeine each day (more than eight cups of coffee or tea). Some women find it easy to reduce the quantity, others prefer to change to decaffeinated drinks, others to stop drinking caffeine-containing liquids. Some women feel that they need coffee and drink two cups to 'get started' in the morning. Coffee drinking is also a social event when a woman meets with her friends. If she doesn't join in she may feel uncomfortable and an 'outsider'. The aim should be to reduce the amount of caffeine ingested in a way that doesn't interfere with the woman's life style too much, and not to make the woman feel guilty about drinking any coffee or tea.

In the health check-up the question of smoking tobacco should be raised. Although in the past 10 years fewer adult women are smoking, tobacco-induced lung cancer is increasing among middle-aged women. Unfortunately tobacco is an addictive drug and many people find it difficult to break the habit. A cigarette may be a solace in moments of stress. However, as there is some evidence that in some women hot flushes may be aggravated by cigarette smoking, the menopausal years may be a time when it is easier to break the addiction.

The general health check-up should lead to a discussion with the health professional about the specific symptoms that are affecting the woman. As we noted in Chapter 7, hot flushes and a dry or painful vagina are the only confirmed physical symptoms associated with the menopause. If the hot flush occurs at night, when a woman is in bed, well insulated by bedclothes, the raised body temperature during the flush may cause her to sweat and to wake up. If she does she may find it difficult to go to sleep again. In other words, she develops insomnia. But if the hot flushes are relieved by treatment, the night sweats and the insomnia will also be relieved.

## HORMONE (OESTROGEN) REPLACEMENT TREATMENT OR HRT

Hormone replacement treatment (HRT), is sometimes called oestrogen replacement treatment, as the lack of oestrogen which follows the menopause is the main cause of the major symptoms occurring after the menopause. Oestrogen relieves the hot flushes and the dry vagina and, if taken for a number of years, reduces the likelihood of heart attack and prevents osteoporosis. (Osteoporosis is discussed in Chapter 10 and heart disease in Chapter 11.)

In recent years, it has become evident that if the woman has not had a hysterectomy, oestrogen given alone may overstimulate the lining of the uterus and lead, in a few cases, to the development of a cancer of the lining of the uterus (endometrial cancer). A woman is protected against this cancer if she takes another hormone, a progestogen, for about 12 days each month. As the woman takes two female sex hormones, the preferred term is hormone replacement treatment.

Oestrogen is usually prescribed as tablets to be taken by mouth. Some women prefer to obtain the oestrogen through the skin by applying an oestradiol patch or rubbing in an oestrogen gel, whilst others prefer an oestradiol implant. Other women, particularly if they have a dry or painful vagina, prefer to use an oestrogen (usually oestriol) vaginal cream or a vaginal tablet (pessary), to relieve the vaginal symptoms.

Oestrogen treatment has to be adjusted to suit each woman, as different women require different doses of oestrogen to relieve the symptoms of hot flushes, and to avoid the side effects of tender or enlarged breasts.

As well as providing oestrogen and progestogen tablets, some pharmaceutical companies provide packs of tablets containing both oestrogen tablets and tablets containing oestrogen and a progestogen. These 'combination preparations' are found to be more convenient by some women.

With all these choices a woman should talk to her doctor or other health professional, if she wants to learn about the most appropriate way for her to use hormone replacement.

### Which hormone to use?

As oestrogen is the mainstay of treatment, oestrogen preparations are available which, as mentioned, can be taken by mouth, absorbed through the skin, through the vagina, or implanted into the tissue under the skin. As well, a new preparation which has oestrogenic, progestogen and androgenic properties is available and can be taken by mouth. This preparation is called Livial, and, as mentioned, combination preparations are also available (Table 8.1).

The oestrogen preparations are (1) synthetic oestrogens; (2) equine oestrogens and (3) the so-called 'natural' oestrogens.

The two synthetic oestrogens currently used in treatment of the menopause are ethinyl oestradiol and its derivative, mestranol. The synthetic oestrogens are absorbed rapidly into the body but

**Table 8.1:** Hormone preparations currently available for the treatment of menopausal symptoms, the prevention of osteoporosis and the reduction in risk of heart attack

| Preparation | Trade name | Dose per day |
|---|---|---|
| *Oral preparations* | | |
| Equine oestrogens | Premarin | 0.3–2.5 mg |
| 'Natural' oestrogens | | |
|   Estropipate | Ogen, Harmogen | 0.625–2.0 mg |
|   Oestradiol valerate | Progynova | 1.0–2.0 mg |
|   Oestradiol (micronized) | Estace | 1.0–2.0 mg |
|   Oestriol | Ovestin | 1.0–4.0 mg |
| Synthetic oestrogens | | |
|   Ethinyl oestradiol | Estigen; Feminone; Lynoral: Primogen | 0.01–0.03 mg |
| Tibolone | Livial | 2.5 mg |
| *Combined oral preparations* | | |
| Equine oestrogens and norgestrel | Prempak | 1 tablet of oestrogen daily and an additional 1 tablet of norgestrel from day 17–28 of each month |
| Oestradiol valerate and levonorgestrel | Cycloprogynova | 1 tablet daily for 21 days |
| Oestradiol valerate and cyproterone acetate | Climen | " |
| Oestradiol, oestriol and norethisterone acetate | Kliogest | " |
| *Trasdermal oestrogens* | Estraderm patch | 0.05–0.1 mg The patch is changed every 4 days |
| *Percutaneous oestrogen* | Oestrogel | 1.5 mg rubbed into an area of the skin each day |
| *Vaginal preparations* | Ovestin ovules Kolpon pesssaries | 1 daily, reducing to 1 twice a week |
| | Dienoestrol cream Ovestin cream Premarin cream | Fill applicator to mark and insert into vagina each day, or 2 to 3 times a week |

metabolize (break-down) slowly and with difficulty; they stimulate liver enzymes more than do the oestrogens of the other two groups.

The equine oestrogens (also known as conjugated equine oestrogens) are derived from the urine of mares, and in this sense they are natural. The principal hormone in equine oestrogens is equilin, which is not made by humans and has no biological effect in a woman's body, but there is sufficient amount of oestradiol in the substance to make conjugated equine oestrogens a useful product.

The so-called natural oestrogens, although made in the laboratory, are called 'natural' because their metabolism is very similar to that of oestrogens produced by the body.

With several oestrogen preparations available (Table 8.1), a woman and her doctor might reasonably ask: 'Which oestrogen preparation is the safest and the most effective?' The drug manufacturers naturally want doctors to believe that their product is superior to any of the others available, that it is the safest and that it produces the fewest undesirable side-effects. Drug manufacturers research their new drugs in a responsible way and the research is controlled by government institutions, to make sure that the new drug is as safe as it is humanly possible to be.

In studying the effects on the body of oestrogen preparations, the pharmaceutical manufacturers have looked at very many biochemical and metabolic changes that occur in a woman's body. In collaboration with doctors, they have investigated the prevalence of the undesirable side-effects in their product. This research is of immense value and importance but the results are often interpreted by the sales division of the pharmaceutical company in ways that are rather devious. This is understandable, as the manufacturers invest a large amount of money in developing a new product to the stage at which it is available to treat a condition. Unless they can recoup their investment they are likely to go out of business.

If the voluminous medical literature regarding the available oestrogen preparations is scrutinized carefully and critically, there is surprisingly little difference between the biochemical and metabolic effects of the various preparations, provided the dose of each oestrogen is equivalent (equipotent) (Table 8.2). There is also surprisingly little difference between their undesirable side-effects.

A possible exception to this is that ethinyl oestradiol is broken down (metabolized) in the body more slowly than the so-called 'natural' oestrogens, so that its effect lasts longer. Because of this,

**Table 8.2:** Equivalent doses of various oestrogen preparations, taken by mouth, to relieve menopausal symptoms

| | |
|---|---|
| Ethinyl oestradiol | 0.01 mg (10 mg) |
| Conjugated equine oestrogens | 0.625 mg |
| Piperazine oestrone sulphate | 0.625 mg |
| Oestradiol valerate | 2.0 mg |
| Oestriol hemisuccinate | 4.0 mg |

ethinyl oestradiol (and to a lesser extent conjugated equine oestrogens) may alter certain liver enzymes and perhaps liver function. In contrast, the 'natural' oestrogens have only a small effect on liver function. But whether or not these changes of liver function are important clinically is not clear.

Some doctors believe that an alteration in liver function predisposes to high blood pressure, to gall bladder disease, to high blood lipid levels and to an increased ability of the blood to clot. This may cause a clot to form in a vein (thrombosis). More rarely, a clot may detach and reach the lungs, causing a pulmonary embolus. Other doctors believe that the alteration in liver function is an interesting observation but has little clinical significance. They point out that if the changes are dangerous to a woman, the 50 million women taking the contraceptive pill are at risk. This is because the oestrogen used in the pill is ethinyl oestradiol and the dose taken for 21 days every month is higher than that taken each month by menopausal women.

The arguments against this belief are that women taking the pill are younger, so the risk of thrombosis in veins is less, and that the pill contains progestogen (a synthetic form of the hormone, progesterone), which may counteract the effects of oestrogen on blood clotting. However, this argument is invalid as most menopausal women are also prescribed a progestogen, which is usually taken for 10 to 14 days each month.

At present there is no evidence that any one formulation of oestrogen is better than any other in eliminating menopausal symptoms, and it doesn't matter much which one is prescribed. The doctor's preference, the woman's wishes and the cost of the formulation should be assessed, before choosing the oestrogen preparation favoured.

This is demonstrated by the hormones used to help menopausal women in different countries. In the USA, the majority of doctors choose Premarin, given cyclically for 25 days each month, and give the progestogen, Provera, for the last 10 days of each course of treatment to those women who have not had a hysterectomy. In Britain, over half of doctors who treat menopausal women choose the combined oestrogen/progestogen preparation, Prempak; and about a third choose Cycloprogynova. In Australia, increasing numbers of doctors are suggesting that the woman takes either Ogen or Premarin continuously, and takes either Primolut–N or Provera for the first 12 days each month. In Scandinavian countries, the preferred oestrogen is a mixture of oestradiol and oestriol.

A new oestrogen-like preparation has been developed for menopausal symptoms and is available in several countries which may be the preferred choice for many women. It is called Livial. The hormone eliminates menopausal symptoms and after 2 or 3 months use most women cease to have withdrawal bleeds. It does not affect the endometrium adversely (see page 65). It prevents bone loss, so reducing the chance that the woman will develop osteoporosis. It does not alter liver function, blood lipids or blood clotting.

## PROGESTOGENS

During the reproductive years of a woman's life, following ovulation the hormone, progesterone, is produced. Progesterone reduces the stimulating (and perhaps cancer-producing) effects of unopposed oestrogen on the tissues of the genital tract and the breasts.

Synthetic progesterone-like substances — called progestogens — are equally effective in protecting a woman's tissues against the undesirable effects of oestrogen. They have the advantage that they can be given by mouth, while 'natural progesterone' must be given by injection or absorbed from the vagina, although recently a preparation of progesterone that is effective by mouth has been developed.

To protect menopausal women from the most serious undesirable effect of oestrogen treatment, that is, the slightly increased risk of developing a cancer of the endometrium (the lining of the uterus), a progestogen is prescribed to women who have not had a hysterectomy, and to women who have had a hysterectomy because of endometriosis. The reason for prescribing a progestogen to women who have had endometriosis treated by hysterectomy, is because there is a theoretical risk that a cancer may develop in one of tiny deposits of endometriosis which have formed on the surface of the ovaries, or the Fallopian tubes or on other organs in the pelvis.

Most menopausal women who have not had a hysterectomy would be wise to take a progestogen for 12 days each calendar month, although other regimens of treatment are available (see below).

The use of a progestogen in this manner leads to a withdrawal bleed (menstruation), in 85 per cent of women. It usually occurs on the last 2 days of taking the progestogen or just after ceasing to take the hormone. It is usually light and lasts between 3 and 5 days. As the months pass, the bleeding tends to become lighter and ceases in some women.

A bleed earlier in the course of the progestogen indicates that the dose is insufficient to protect the endometrium from oestrogen-induced stimulation, and the dose taken each day for the 12 days should be increased.

The continuation of menstruation distresses many women and may be the reason why some stop taking hormone replacement treatment. Research in Australia, England and The Netherlands shows that 70 per cent of women would prefer not to have the bleeds. For this reason, regimens in which bleeding occurs less often are being investigated. These regimens are discussed on page 73–75

Several types of progestogen are available currently (Table 8.3). Proponents of each claim that their particular progestogen is superior, but in reality there is little difference. In the USA, medroxyprogesterone acetate is preferred, as the product is thought to alter blood lipids less than the others. However, a Swedish study suggests that the difference found is due to the use of a larger than necessary daily dose of norethisterone or levonorgestrel. Some doctors prefer to use one of these two products, as medroxyprogesterone acetate (in the recommended daily dose of 5–10 mg) is less effective in suppressing the oestrogen-induced changes in endometrial cells. New progestogens that have no effect on blood lipids are becoming available (desorgestrel, gestodene and norgestimate). These may replace the older progestogens in the near future.

Apart from the 'withdrawal bleed', the administration of a progestogen (or a 'natural progesterone'), may cause problems in 10

Table 8.3: Progestogens currently available for hormone treatment in the menopausal years

| Name | Trade name | Dose (mg a day) Taken for 12 days each month |
|---|---|---|
| Norethisterone | Primolut-N | 1.0*–2.5 mg |
|  | Micronor | 0.35*–0.70 mg |
| Medroxyprogesterone acetate | Provera | 10 mg |
| Desogestrel |  | 0.125 mg |
| Cyproterone acetate | Androcur | 1 mg |
| Micronized progesterone | Utrogestan | 200 mg |
| Dydrogesterone | Duphaston | 10–20 mg |

\* This dose is usually sufficient to suppress the adverse effect of oestrogen on the uterus and the endometrium.

to 25 per cent of women. In some of these women the progestogen produces feelings of irritability, fatigue or depression. In other women, one or more of the following may occur: abdominal bloating, abdominal cramps, headaches, drowsiness, breast tenderness, and weight gain. The symptoms may vary from month to month, and may resemble those experienced by women who have the premenstrual syndrome.

Although often attributed to progestogen, the cause is more complex as women treated with large doses of progestogen for cancer, do not report the symptoms. It is possible that the *combination* of oestrogen and progesterone is the cause.

In most instances, the symptoms can be managed by adjusting the dose or changing to another progestogen or oestrogen. For example, changing the oestrogen may relieve the negative mood symptoms, as may a change from medroxyprogesterone acetate (Provera), to norethisterone (Primolut-N), or vice versa. There is also some evidence that changing the progestogen may reduce the abdominal bloating and cramps. The new hormonal preparation, Livial, may enable women to avoid the psychological symptoms some get when taking a progestogen.

Investigations are continuing to find ways of relieving these troublesome side effects.

## HOW HORMONE REPLACEMENT TREATMENT IS PRESCRIBED

As we noted earlier, most doctors prescribe oestrogen tablets or capsules, which the woman takes by mouth. A few doctors give oestrogen tablets that are absorbed from the vagina, and a few 'implant' oestrogen tablets under the skin. Recently a new oestrogen preparation has been developed that is absorbed from a 'patch' fixed to the skin.

An advantage of the last three ways of prescribing oestrogen over oestrogens taken by mouth is that oral oestrogens are absorbed from the gut and are first carried to the liver. As has been mentioned, they may induce the production of liver proteins and enzymes. As well, a variable portion of the oestrogen is inactivated in the liver and consequently produces no beneficial effect. The inactivity may be overcome by giving a larger dose of oestrogen or by changing the chemical nature of the oestrogen so that less is inactivated. One way of achieving this is to make the oestrogen particles very small, by 'micronizing' them. This is a process in which the substances are broken down into tiny particles, which are absorbed into the body more easily and are less likely to be inactivated before they have had their effect. Micronized oestrogen can be taken by mouth or placed in the vagina.

If the woman has not had a hysterectomy (or if the hysterectomy was performed because she had endometriosis), she should also take one of the progestogens for 10 to 12 days each month, to protect her from the possibility of developing uterine (endometrial) cancer — as we have discussed.

*Oral oestrogen and progestogens*   There are several regimens for prescribing hormone replacement, each of which has its advocates. It is hard to decide if any one is better than any other (and fashion plays a large part), as little research has taken place to find out what *women* prefer.

- Most doctors in the USA prescribe oestrogen for 21 days a month, and ask the woman to take a progestogen for the last 7 to 14 days of the course. The woman takes no hormones for 7 days, during which time she may have a recurrence of her symptoms, and usually has a withdrawal bleed. After the gap of 7 days, she starts another course. The method is termed *cyclical hormone treatment*.

- Most doctors in Australia recommend that the woman takes an oestrogen tablet every day without a break, and takes a progestogen tablet as well for the first 12 days of each month. During the time when she takes the progestogen, she may expect to have a bleed. Four women in every 5 taking this regimen of treatment will have a 'withdrawal bleed'. If the bleed occurs in the first 10 days of the progesterone treatment, the dose should be increased, as her uterus may not be protected against endometrial cancer. (This also applies to women who choose the cyclical treatment.) If the woman does not bleed, or bleeds on or after day 11 when she is taking the progestogen, her uterus is protected against endometrial cancer, at least to the level at which this cancer occurs among women not taking hormones.

    Oestrogen taken each day (*continuous hormone treatment*), has the benefit that meopausal symptoms are controlled *all* the time, and the time of the withdrawal bleed can be advanced or retarded to suit circumstances.
- Because many women do not like having a withdrawal bleed, and 1 in 15 develops mood changes or bloating (a bit like the changes which occur before a woman's periods), research is underway to see if oestrogen can be given continuously (either by mouth or as a patch), and a progestogen tablet for 12 days *every 3rd month*. If the research shows that this regimen protects the uterus against endometrial cancer as effectively as the other methods, it may be chosen by some women. Early reports of this regimen show that the endometrium is not stimulated.
- Another way of preventing withdrawal bleeds and possibly of reducing the mood changes associated with taking a progestogen intermittently, is to take a tablet of oestrogen and one of progestogen each day. This is *combined continuous hormone replacement treatment*. Several combinations are available which are effective in preventing menopausal symptoms and endometrial stimulation and which inhibit bone loss. The advantage of the method is that most women do not have any bleeds after 3 to 6 months of taking the tablets, although a number of women bleed at irregular, variable times during the first 3 to 4 months of treatment, particularly if the method is used in the first year or two after the menopause. The effects of a progestogen taken daily on the presence of problems such as irritability, headache, bloating and 'fluid retention' are not yet clear and more research is needed.

### A new hormone for HRT

A hormone preparation which has oestrogen, progestogen and slight androgen activity has been developed. Women who do not like taking oestrogen and progestogen tablets may prefer this simple method. The woman takes one tablet of Livial each day. Using Livial, one woman in five may have some irregular bleeding in the first three months, after which the bleeding ceases and the woman ceases to have periods. As with the combined continuous hormone replacement treatment, the use of Livial in the first year or two after the menopause is more likely to be associated with irregular bleeding episodes and women may prefer to delay starting Livial until after this time. Livial protects the endometrium against cancer, does not alter the blood lipids and offers protection against bone loss and the development of osteoporosis.

*Vaginal oestrogen*  Oestrogen tablets or creams placed in the vagina are readily absorbed into the body. An example of this absorption has been reported from Sweden. The scientists found that 0.2 mg of the micronized oestradiol placed in the vagina produced the blood levels of oestrogen found in a woman during the first half of her menstrual cycle. If the micronized oestradiol was given by mouth, ten times the dose was needed to produce the same result.

This means that if oestrogen is given vaginally, the dose must be reduced. Many menopausal women do not like placing tablets or cream in their vagina, so that the vaginal route is usually only chosen if the woman's main complaint is vaginal dryness, burning or discomfort. Of course, the hormone is equally effective for these symptoms if given by one of the other routes, provided the dose is adjusted.

*Vaginal oestrogen ring*  A novel system of giving oestrogen is being studied. This is for the woman to insert a polysiloxane (plastic) ring, about 50 mm (2 ins) in size, high into her vagina. The ring is impregnated with oestrogen, which is released slowly for 2 to 3 months. The woman leaves the ring in her vagina, only taking it out and replacing it at intervals. She can have sexual intercourse with the ring in.

*Transdermal systems of giving oestrogen*  This is a new development which has several advantages. Oestradiol (in a 0.05 or 0.1mg dose) is mixed in a solvent gel and is applied to the skin in a 'plastic' patch, which sticks to the skin (Fig. 8.1). The oestrogen is absorbed through the skin and enters the blood circulation. Oestrogen patches

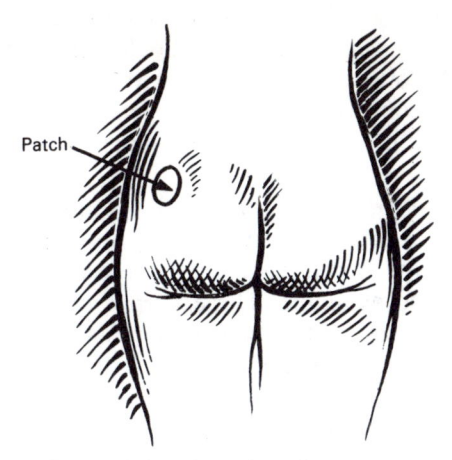

**Figure 8.1:** Transdermal oestrogen

are stuck to the skin on the woman's abdomen or between her buttocks, and are peeled off and replaced every 3 or 4 days on a different part of the skin.

Unfortunately, one woman in six in northern Europe and the USA develops redness under the patch. Some of these women also complain of itchiness under the patch and a few develop small blisters. These changes are minor in most of the affected women, but in 3 per cent cause problems, which persuades the woman to change to another way of obtaining hormone replacement.

In countries with hot and humid climates, up to half of women using patches develop skin redness, and many of them have itchy skins, and one woman in 20 develops small blisters under the patch, which limits their use in these countries.

The lower dose of oestrogen is chosen first. The woman keeps a record of the number of hot flushes she experiences each day. If the number has not fallen to less than two a day in 2 weeks, the dose of oestrogen is doubled.

*Percutaneous oestrogen* This system of giving oestrogen is popular in France and is being used by women in some other countries. Like oestrogen from patches, percutaneous oestrogen gel enters the peripheral blood directly, giving very stable circulating levels in the blood, and avoiding passage through the liver.

The woman rubs a small amount of the oestradiol gel (Oestrogel 1.5–3.0 mg) on to the upper arms and shoulders each day, rather like applying a body lotion. The gel dries within 2 to 3 minutes. It is claimed that in contrast to oestradiol patches, no skin reactions result from percutaneous oestrogen treatment.

*Oestrogen injections and 'implants'* A few women prefer to have an injection of a 'long acting oestrogen' every 3 to 4 weeks. 'Pellets' of oestrogen, which are implanted under the skin about every 6 months (Fig. 8.2), are also available. These preparations release a small quantity of oestrogen into the woman's circulation each day so that the she does not have to remember to take a daily tablet or to place a 'patch' on her skin every 3 or 4 days.

Usually, the slow steady release of the oestrogen maintains the blood level of oestradiol which relieves the woman's symptoms over a period of months. As the implant becomes smaller, the supply of oestrogen drops to a level at which symptoms recur. When this happens, a further implant is needed. Because the relief of the symptoms depends not only on the quantity of circulating oestrogen, but on theability of the woman's cells to absorb the hormone, the time of the return of the symptoms differs in different women.

Paradoxically, a few women (probably less than 1 per cent of all women who have chosen an implant) develop troublesome symptoms at a time when the level of oestrogen in their blood is still high — when measured by laboratory tests. At present, there is some concern as the amount of circulating oestrogen, measured by different blood tests, varies very considerably, so that some women who are found to have a high blood level of oestrogen may not really have one. This problem is being researched at present.

If the blood measurements accurately represent the situation, women who have these high blood levels of oestrogen usually have been using implants for a number of years. In a few cases, the blood oestrogen level may be above that reached at the time of the oestrogen peak during the menstrual cycle. If the woman does not have a uterus, this should cause no problem, although the high oestrogen level may cause breast tenderness of a few women. A woman who has not had a hysterectomy and ceases to use oestrogen replacement needs to continue to take a progestogen (12 days a month), until the blood level of oestrogen has dropped to that found after the menopause, because the persisting high plasma level may stimulate the endometrium unduly.

HOW TO MANAGE THE MENOPAUSE

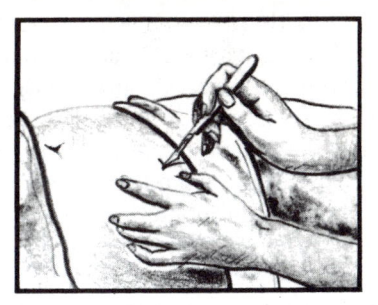

Under a local anaesthetic a small incision is made through the skin of the abdomen

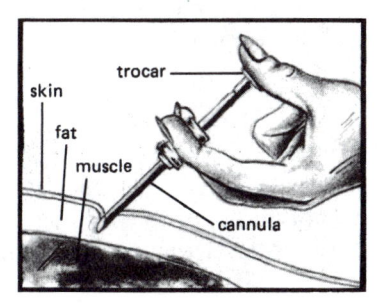

A trocar and cannula are pushed through the incision into the tissue between the skin and the muscle; the trocar is then withdrawn

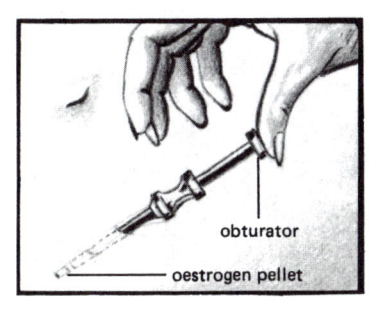

The hormone pellet is injected into the tissue through the cannula

Figure 8.2:  Oestrogen (oestradiol) implant

These findings suggest that women who choose implants should have an accurate blood test made to check the level of oestrogen when symptoms return, before a new implant is inserted. If the level of oestrogen in the blood is high, in spite of menopausal symptoms, the woman and her doctor will have to decide whether or not to insert another implant. If the woman choses not to have a further implant, she may choose another method of oestrogen replacement, preferably by the transdermal or the vaginal route, rather than suffering from menopausal symptoms while waiting for the oestrogen level in the blood to drop to the normal postmenopausal range.

A few doctors add the male hormone, testosterone, to the oestrogen implant claiming that the testosterone improves the muscle tone of postmenopausal women and increases their sexual desire and responsiveness (see Chapter 14).

### Effectiveness of hormone replacement treatment

The most obvious way to judge the effectiveness of oestrogen treatment is that the hot flushes or the burning feeling in the vagina cease or are much reduced. However, a way of determining the

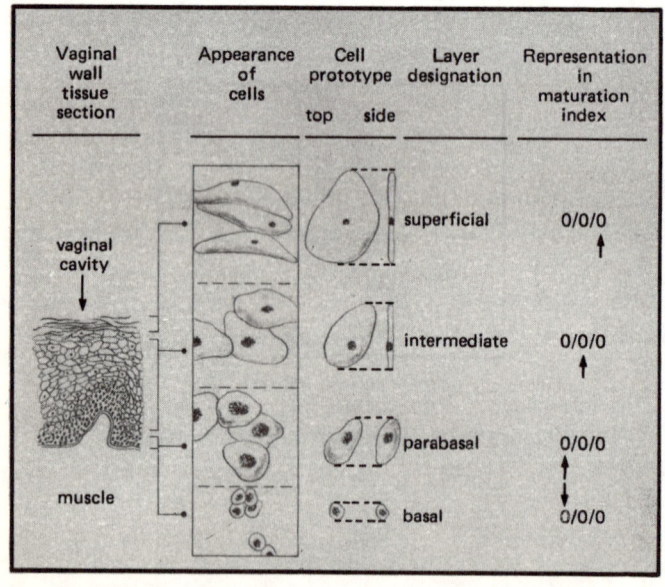

Figure 8.3: Maturation of cells in the vaginal mucosa

effectiveness of treatment was (and is) used by many doctors, particularly in Europe and the USA, who claim it is more 'scientific'. The method is to calculate the 'maturity index' of the vaginal epithelium. The thickness of the vaginal wall can be deduced from the type of vaginal cells shed into the vaginal cavity. The proponents of this method believe the appearance and number of the various cells show the degree of oestrogen circulating in the woman's body. It is true that development or maturation of the vaginal epithelium depends on the level of circulating oestrogen, but once a quantum of oestrogen is circulating, the relationship ceases.

Despite this, many doctors believe that a vaginal swab should be taken from all menopausal women to help plan treatment and at intervals when the woman is receiving oestrogen to check the effectiveness of treatment. The swab is smeared onto a slide, stained and examined through a microscope. The slide shows the types of cells that make up the vaginal wall in differing proportions (Fig. 8.3).

By counting the proportion of each cell type in the smear, a 'maturation index' is obtained. The higher the proportion of parabasal cells, the greater the need for treatment; the higher the proportion of superficial cells, the greater the effect of oestrogen. Recent studies have shown that this test is of little or no value in determining the dose required or the duration of oestrogen treatment. It has no place in the management of the menopause.

### Investigations needed before taking hormone replacement treatment

As in any medical procedure, the doctor should take a history enquiring about general health, high blood pressure, diabetes, smoking habits, exercise and so on. A physical examination, including a vaginal examination is essential.

Until recently, many menopausal women had their uterus curetted under an anaesthetic to remove the entire endometrial lining. Alternatively, a specimen of the uterine lining was taken without an anaesthetic. This procedure is called an endometrial biopsy, and involves the insertion of a small tube into the uterus to extract a piece of the endometrium, which can then be examined microscopically to make sure that there is no abnormality in the cells. Recent experience has shown that if the woman is given oestrogen, and progestogen for at least 12 days each month, the procedure is not required nor justified.

A few American physicians give a small dose of a progestogen

**Table 8.4:** Contra-indications to oestrogen treatment

Women who have or have had the following illnesses should not be prescribed oestrogen:
* Acute liver disease
* Chronic liver disease with impaired function
* Breast cancer (but see text)
* A history of two or more episodes of a *recent* acute deep venous thrombosis

Women who have or have had the following illnesses may take oestrogen but require frequent checks:
* High blood pressure
* Diabetes
* Benign breast disease
* Uterine 'fibroids'
* Migraine
* Gall bladder disease
* Chronic thrombophlebitis
* Endometriosis
* Familial high blood lipids

(medroxyprogesterone acetate 10 mg) for 5 days before starting oestrogen treatment. If no bleeding occurs within 7 days of the progestogen, treatment is started. However, if bleeding occurs, an endometrial biopsy is made, although cancer is rarely found (1 in 1000 times).

Most women can safely be prescribed oestrogen treatment after checking that (1) the breasts have no lumps; (2) the blood pressure is normal; (3) there is no enlargement of the internal genital organs; (4) there is no history of irregular bleeding from the uterus.

Certain women should not be prescribed oestrogen for the reasons listed in Table 8.4 but the prohibition is not absolute and if the woman's history discloses that she has had or has one of them she should seek the opinion of her doctor, and may wish for a second opinion. For example, a matter of concern is a history of clotting in a deep vein (thrombosis) or a pulmonary thromboembolism following an operation or childbirth. In the past, this was thought to be a contra-indication to hormone replacement, but this opinion has now changed. If the thrombosis occurred during the time that the woman was menstruating regularly and had not occurred after the woman had recently started taking the Pill, there is no reason why she should not take hormone replacement treatment.

In Table 8.4, breast cancer is stated to be a contra-indication. This is logical as some breast cancers are 'oestrogen dependent'. However, some women who have had breast cancer may have such severe menopausal symptoms, which have not responded to non-hormonal treatments, that life has become intolerable. These women may improve their quality of life considerably if they take hormonal treatment, provided they know that the oestrogen *may* cause the cancer to spread. They should talk about this with their doctor, but ultimately their choice must be respected by the doctor.

Women who have had their ovaries removed in the treatment of cancer of the ovaries may take hormone replacement treatment, as it does not adversely affect the growth or recurrence of the cancer, and relieves some unpleasant menopausal symptoms.

## Principles regarding hormone replacement treatment

There is no doubt that oestrogens will relieve a woman's menopausal symptoms dramatically. This statement applies particularly to the 'cascade' of hot flushes → night sweats → insomnia, and to the vaginal symptoms. Some studies claim that oestrogens improve the mental ability of a menopausal woman (see Chapter 13). Oestrogens are also of great benefit in preventing bone loss in the decade after the menopause, thus preventing osteoporosis (see Chapter 10).

So that the undesirable side-effects of oestrogen are minimized, the following principles should be understood by the woman and her doctor:

- oestrogen should be taken in the lowest effective dose

- if the woman has not had a hysterectomy, a progestogen should be taken with oestrogen at periodic intervals (currently 12 to 14 days each month) to protect the woman against possible uterine (endometrial) cancer

- with this treatment, over 60 per cent of menopausal women will have monthly 'periods' — these are usually scanty and last about 3 days

- provided the bleeds are regular, no concern need be expressed, but if the bleeding becomes irregular in duration or onset, it is likely that the woman's doctor will recommend investigation

- in general, the combination of oestrogen with other hormones or drugs is unnecessary — the exception being a progestogen and occasionally testosterone.

Adherence by the woman, on the advice of her doctor, to these guidelines, makes oestrogen treatment an appropriate and effective method of controlling hot flushes. She is asked to record how many times a day the hot flushes occur, and if the frequency has not fallen to below five after 7 days of treatment, she doubles the dose of oestrogen, taking two tablets each day instead of one. The dose may need to be increased a further step before control is obtained. Some of the pharmaceutical manufacturers are aware of this and provide tablets of different strengths.

The correct dose of progestogen is also important. Too little is ineffective; too much increases the chance of side effects.

The available progestogens are shown in Table 8.3 on page 71. To avoid side-effects, the lowest dose should be given initially. If this leads to a bleed each month on or after the 11th day of taking the progestogen the dose is adequate. If bleeding occurs before day 11, the dose is insufficient to make sure that the endometrium is not being unduly stimulated and the dose should be doubled.

Other possible treatments

Is there any treatment for hot flushes in women who cannot take oestrogens?

Two other forms of treatment for hot flushes are available, although neither is as effective as oestrogen in relieving the symptoms. The first is to use a drug normally prescribed to reduce high blood pressure. The drug is called clonidine (Dixarit). Clonidine reduces the responsiveness of blood vessels, so that they dilate less readily. As vasodilatation precedes a hot flush, its control reduces the frequency of the symptom. Clonidine is more effective if given in the form of a skin patch (transdermal system).

The second treatment is for the woman to take one of two progestogen drugs, either norethisterone (5 mg daily) or medroxyprogesterone (Provera) 10 to 20 mg daily. Either of these hormones seems to reduce the frequency of hot flushes, by half to three-quarters, but does not eliminate them as effectively as oestrogen.

## WHY IS HORMONE REPLACEMENT TREATMENT NOT ACCEPTED BY ALL MENOPAUSAL WOMEN?

As mentioned earlier in this book, about 25 per cent of women in most countries have no symptoms in the menopausal years, and in a further 35 per cent, the symptoms are so mild that the woman does not visit a doctor. In most developed countries, many of these women (and many more in the developing countries), either do not know about the value of hormone replacement or fear that the hormones may damage their body. In the USA, rather more menopausal women visit their doctor for menopausal problems. However, even in countries where about 70 per cent of menopausal women seek medical help, and are prescribed hormone treatment for menopausal symptoms, over half either do not take the prescribed hormones or only take them sporadically. It has been estimated that in these countries fewer than 20 per cent of women are taking hormone replacement at any one time, and of more concern, fewer than 10 per cent of menopausal women are taking the hormone treatment regularly for the 10 (or more) years recommended for protection against osteoporosis and heart disease.

As women grow older, particularly after the age of 60, increasingly fewer continue to take hormone replacement treatment, yet women of this age have a higher chance of developing heart disease, for which hormone replacement treatment offers some degree of protection (see page 122). There is also evidence that oestrogen continued into old age reduces the risk of osteoporotic fractures.

The question is, why do so few women take hormone replacement

Table 8.5: Some problems associated with hormone treatment and their solutions

| | |
|---|---|
| The symptoms are not relieved | The dose of the hormones needs to be increased |
| The breasts become very tender and/or painful | Reduce the dose of the oestrogen |
| Symptoms of irritability, mood upsets are severe | Reduce the dose of the progestogen |
| The 'withdrawal bleed' is heavy | Try reducing the amount of oestrogen, or increasing the amount of progestogen |

**Table 8.6:** Common misconceptions about oestrogen in the menopause

| | |
|---|---|
| Not 'natural' | Taking oestrogen is as natural as taking any other endocrine (hormone) substance when a deficiency is present in the body |
| Makes the periods come back | For most women this is true, but treatments are being devised to stop them returning |
| Causes heavy periods | If a progestogen is taken the bleed is usually light and predictable |
| Causes cancer | Oestrogen does not cause breast cancer, and its effect on the uterus can be eliminated by taking progestogens |
| Causes weight gain | Oestrogen may lead to some fat being deposited on the hips and thighs, but it does not cause weight gain if the dose given is in the usual range |
| Hormones are only needed if you have menopausal symptoms | Oestrogen taken regularly will delay the onset of osteoporosis and may reduce the chance of having a heart attack |
| HRT alters your blood cholesterol and blood lipids unfavourably | Oestrogen lowers the blood cholesterol and increases the level of the 'good' cholesterol, HDL. The progestogens now used in the doses prescribed do not prevent this from happening. |

treatment? The first reason is that many women have misconceptions about oestrogen. In Table 8.5 and Table 8.6 some of the most often voiced misconceptions are shown and the answer to the misconception is given. Other women start taking the hormones and then stop because of side-effects, particularly bleeding problems.

The problem may be reduced if women can talk with a health professional and their anxieties and concerns can be discussed openly. A study in the USA (of a small selected number of women) showed that when this happened, over 80 per cent of women continued taking the hormones regularly.

# APPENDIX

Oestrogen metabolism

Some readers may wish to know more about the way in which the oestrogens are metabolized in the body; this appendix will help them to understand the processes.

In the body, three main oestrogens circulate. They are: *oestradiol*, which is the most active form; *oestrone*, which is less active; and *oestriol*, which is a relatively very weak oestrogen.

Oestradiol is synthesized in the ovaries and enters the blood bound to a carrier protein. It is carried to certain 'target' cells, which have 'receptors' and bind onto the oestrogen. It is then absorbed into the target cells.

In the target cell, oestradiol is converted into oestrone, a less active oestrogen, which is transferred to the nucleus of the cell where it alters the cell's processes through a complicated series of changes.

Oestrone is kept in store in the body as oestrone sulphate, and is also the form in which oestrogens are excreted from the body. There are several chemical pathways by which oestrone is metabolized. A major pathway converts oestrone into oestriol. This oestrogen was thought to be relatively inactive biologically, but it is now known that if it is given over a period of time it has biological effects similar to those of oestradiol and oestrone.

Two other metabolic pathways are also biologically important. In the first, oestrone is converted into 2-hydroxyoestrone. This substance is a catecholoestrogen and is probably the biological form in which oestrogen is taken up by, and is active in, the brain. It is also the major breakdown product of oestradiol found in the urine. In the second of these pathways oestrone is metabolized into 4-hydroxyoestrone. This substance binds easily to oestrogen receptors in tissues (although not as easily as oestradiol and 2-hydroxyoestrone), but its biological actions have not yet been clarified.

## EFFECTS OF OESTROGENS ON THE LIVER

The several types of oestrogens available to treat the menopause (see Table 8.1) may be given by mouth, by injection, absorbed from the vagina or given through the skin. If they are given by mouth, the oestrogen is absorbed from the gut and carried to the liver, as over 90 per cent of blood that has supplied the gut passes through the liver. If oestrogens are given by injection, absorbed through the vagina or given through the skin, the effects on the liver are minimized, as only 10 per cent of the blood passes through the liver. By avoiding having to pass through the liver, the ratio of oestradiol to oestrone in the blood becomes much more like the ratio that occurs in a woman's body in the years before the menopause. However, as mentioned, oestrone sulphate, and conjugated equine oestrogen have to pass through the liver before they become biologically active, so there is no benefit in giving either of these drugs except by mouth.

Each type of synthetic oestrogen affects liver function in a different way.

*Ethinyl oestradiol* This oestrogen is readily absorbed from the gut when taken by mouth, and is carried to the liver. The liver cells preferentially take up twice the amount of ethinyl oestradiol compared with that taken up by the uterus. This means that the amount of ethinyl oestradiol in the liver will be at least twice that in any other organ irrespective of its route of administration. Ethinyl oestradiol is also metabolized slowly so that its effect on liver function is greater than that of the other synthetic oestrogens.

*'Natural' oestrogens* The effect of the so-called 'natural' oestrogens on liver function depends on the route of administration and on the type of oestrogen. *Piperazine oestrone sulphate* (estropipate), for example, is only effective when taken by mouth, because the piperazine portion blocks the biological function of the oestrone until it is removed. Piperazine is added to enhance absorption of the compound from the gut and is removed in the liver. After its removal, oestrone sulphate, which is also an inert oestrogen, remains. Liver enzymes remove the sulphate leaving the active oestrone.

*Conjugated equine oestrogen* This is obtained from the urine of pregnant mares. It is a mixture of oestrogens — 65 per cent being oestrone sulphate and 35 per cent is equilin, an oestrogen not found in humans. As with piperazine oestrone sulphate, it has to pass through the liver to have the sulphate removed and become biologically active. In the liver, conjugated equine oestrogens induce liver protein production, to a greater extent than do the so-called 'natural' oestrogens, but less than does ethinyl oestradiol. Premarin has been called a natural oestrogen, but it is not. It is a natural oestrogen in horses, not humans!

*Oestradiol valerate*   This compound is absorbed readily because of the valerate which, on reaching the liver, is removed, leaving active oestradiol.

*Micronized oestradiol*   This form of oestradiol is readily absorbed because of the 'micro' size of its particles. It then passes through the liver on its way to target cells without being further altered.

*Oestriol*   Oestriol is also available to treat menopausal symptoms, It is a weak oestrogen and large doses are needed.

# 9
# THE SIDE-EFFECTS OF HORMONAL TREATMENT

Oestrogens are hormones; they enter cells that have special areas on their surface (receptors) enabling the hormone to 'bind' to the cell. The cells that have the largest number of receptors for oestrogen are those of the genital tract and the breast milk-ducts. Inside the cells, oestrogen is transferred to the nucleus of the cell where it stimulates cell growth. In this way oestrogen may interfere with the normal life of the cell and may possibly promote cancer in tissues that have many oestrogen receptors, such as the lining of the uterus and the glandular tissues of the breasts.

Oestrogen is secreted by the ovaries throughout a woman's fertile years, that is from about 13 to 50 years of age, but endometrial cancer and breast cancer are uncommon during these years. The reason that cancer is unusual is because the second female sex hormone, progesterone, which is also secreted by the ovary, controls and counteracts the stimulating effect of oestrogen.

## CANCER OF THE ENDOMETRIUM

The possible cancer-producing effect of oestrogen was not recognized in the 1960s and 1970s, when many menopausal women were prescribed oestrogen tablets to help them remain 'forever feminine'. Then in 1975, three reports produced evidence that oestrogen taken in this way, without taking a progestogen as well to 'oppose' the oestrogen led to endometrial cancer in a number of women. A woman taking oestrogen daily for 3 or 4 years had three times the chance of developing endometrial cancer compared with a woman not taking oestrogen. The actual risk increased from 1 per 1000 women to 3 per 1000 women. These findings were disputed by many doctors at the time and a controversy followed. But they have been shown to be correct. Since 1975, seventeen carefully conducted studies have been made, all but one of which have confirmed that unopposed oestrogen treatment is associated with an increased risk that the woman will develop endometrial cancer, but if she does, the cancer is usually curable by surgery.

The results of these investigations and the concern that oestrogen treatment might be dangerous has led to a change in the hormonal treatment of the menopause. It is now current medical practice for menopausal women who have the symptoms of hot flushes (and the 'cascade' symptoms of night sweats and insomnia) or a painful vagina and who are taking oestrogen, to take, in addition, a small dose of progestogen for 12 days each month. This regimen effectively prevents oestrogen stimulating the endometrial cells unduly. The woman has no increased risk of developing endometrial cancer compared with women of a similar age who do not take oestrogens.

There is a problem. Over 90 per cent of women who take the oestrogen–progestogen combination will have a 'withdrawal' bleed (usually scanty and lasting 3–4 days) during the treatment-free week, or during the time they are taking the progestogen. These 'periods' may annoy some women who had hoped that their menstrual periods would cease with the menopause. The advantage of having a withdrawal bleed is that it is a useful sign that the endometrium is not being stimulated excessively by oestrogen. If the bleed occurs before the 11th day of the oestrogen–progestogen combination, the dose of progestogen needs to be increased. If it occurs on or after the 11th day, it indicates that the risk of endometrial cancer developing is negligible.

Some doctors believe, as an added precaution to make sure that cancer does not develop, that any woman receiving oestrogen treatment should have a sample of the endometrium (a biopsy) taken every year. This can be done without an anaesthetic by introducing a narrow plastic instrument into the uterus and extracting a piece of the endometrium. Most women who have had the procedure done say the discomfort is slight, but about 20 per cent of women find it painful and 15 per cent find it very painful. The degree of pain and discomfort is reduced if the woman is given a capsule of mefenamic acid (Ponstan) half an hour before the procedure is made. An alternative is to admit the woman to hospital and curette her uterus under a general anaesthetic. This is costly, invasive, and time-consuming.

Doctors who do not recommend an annual endometrial biopsy have several reasons for this. First, fewer than one woman in every 1000 in this age group develops endometrial cancer. Based on routine sampling of menopausal women, it was found that over half of those women in whom cancer was diagnosed had symptoms. In other words, they had irregular bleeding before curettage. This means that to detect one endometrial cancer in those women who have no symptoms, over 2000 endometrial biopsies would have to be made. Second, as progestogen is now given routinely, the possible cancer-producing effect of oestrogen is inhibited. Thus *routine* endometrial curettage is not required, but if a woman taking oestrogen treatment develops irregular, unscheduled bleeding, investigations are essential. The doctor may suggest that she has an ultrasound picture made of her uterus using a vaginal probe. This instrument which is smaller than a vaginal speculum is inserted high into the woman's vagina. The ultrasound picture shows the uterus clearly. The thickness of the endometrium is measured, and if it is in the normal range, endometrial cancer is unlikely to be present.

Other doctors believe it is better to inspect the inside of the uterus with a hysteroscope and remove a sample of the endometrium for examination by a pathologist to be sure that there is no cancer.

Alternatively, the specimen may be obtained by the endometrial biopsy instrument mentioned earlier.

## BREAST CANCER

The question whether oestrogen treatment increases a woman's chance of developing breast cancer is very important because the growth of many forms of breast cancer seem to be increased by oestrogen, and breast cancer is one of the more common cancers in older women affecting one woman in 14, usually after she has reached the menopause.

This concern has led to over 10 well-designed investigations of large numbers of women. The current consensus is that a woman who takes oestrogen for more than 5 years to treat her menopausal symptoms and to prevent osteoporosis increases the risk slightly that she will develop breast cancer compared with a woman who does not take oestrogen. If the woman using HRT has not had a hysterectomy, and takes a progestogen intermittently to avoid developing cancer of the endometrium, her risk of developing breast cancer appears to be increased rather more than if she only took oestrogen. Again the effect is only observed after using HRT for more than 5 years. The reason for the increased risk when a progestogen is taken as well as an oestrogen, appears to be that progestogen, whilst *preventing* proliferation of the endometrial cells, *increases* the proliferation of cells in the ducts of the breasts which have been stimulated by oestrogen.

These findings are preliminary, and further studies are needed to clarify the situation. However, it has been calculated that long-term HRT will delay the onset of osteoporosis and will prevent four deaths from heart disease for each death from breast cancer. Meanwhile the advice given in Chapter 11 for all women in their middle years should be taken. This is that a woman should examine her breasts each month to make sure that no lump has developed and should have an annual breast check from an experienced doctor and a mammogram taken each year from the age of 50. If she follows this advice, should a breast cancer develop almost certainly it will be small and curable.

## CARDIOVASCULAR DISEASE

Four times as many men as women under the age of 50 die from heart attacks. This suggests that in some way oestrogens protect women from cardiovascular disease. Evidence is accumulating that oestrogen taken regularly for years, and the other strategies mentioned on p. 128 reduce the chance that a woman will have a heart attack.

### Thrombosis

Several studies made in the 1970s, have shown that the risk of venous thrombosis and pulmonary embolism is increased among women taking oestrogen-containing compounds. However, the dose of oestrogen given was much larger than that commonly required to control menopausal symptoms. Among menopausal women taking oestrogens or oestrogen–progestogen combinations, most investigators have found no alteration in the blood factors that lead to blood clotting, whichever oestrogen preparation is prescribed, provided the dose was equivalent (equipotent). Clinical experience in the use of oestrogens to treat menopausal symptoms for long periods of time indicates that such treatment is not associated with an increase in deep vein thrombosis.

## HIGH BLOOD PRESSURE

In a small number of women, hormone replacement treatment provokes a rise in blood pressure, so that the woman develops hypertension. If the woman stops treatment, the blood pressure falls to within the normal range. The rise in blood pressure is probably due to the fact that some women's blood vessels are particularly sensitive to the effects of oestrogen and, more probably, to certain of the progestogens. This effect is mediated by enzymes which oestrogen and some progestogens induce the liver cells to synthesize. The new generation progestogens do not have this effect on blood vessels and where they are available should be chosen.

If a woman who is taking hormones develops a high blood pressure, her doctor will stop the treatment for about two weeks, so that the hypertension can be brought under control. After this time the woman may resume taking hormones. Oestrogen given via the vagina or by the transdermal system is to be preferred as it goes straight into the blood stream, and does not cause hypertension. The chance of developing hypertension is one of the reasons why a menopausal woman should see her doctor every year, so that her blood pressure, her breasts and her cervix may be checked.

## GALL BLADDER DISEASE

The incidence of gall bladder disease is increased slightly among women who take oestrogen for long periods to relieve menopausal symptoms. The increase is small and other factors such as obesity and diet are more significant.

## MOOD SYMPTOMS

As noted earlier, women who have not had a hysterectomy are usually prescribed a progestogen for 12 days each month. During the time the woman takes the progestogen, between 15 and 20 per cent develop negative mood changes, becoming irritable, fatiqued, less responsive and sometimes aggressive. These symptoms are similar to those which occur in the premenstrual syndome. The negative mood changes may be mild or quite severe.

If the woman is severely incommoded, the progestogen should be changed (see Table 8.3 page 71) or Livial chosen as the preferred form of HRT.

# 10

# OSTEOPOROSIS

---

*Osteoporosis is an example of a disease that may be preventable in many women if physicians and the public were better informed.*
G Donald Whedon:
*New England Journal of Medicine* 1981

As a woman grows older, her bones become more brittle, and more likely to collapse or fracture. The most common bones first to collapse are those of the vertebrae, which make up the spine. In fact, the collapse is preceded by tiny fractures in the bone. These small fractures are usually painless, although if the process goes on for some time, a whole vertebra may collapse, becoming wedge shaped instead of cube shaped. This leads to the decrease in the person's height that is often observed among older women. About one woman in ten loses one-fifth of her height between the age of 50 and 70 years (Fig 10.1). The most common fractures that occur later, in older people, are those of the wrist and the hip joint. This is because these bones have to carry the most weight if a person slips or falls. A fracture is an acute, painful event, which needs immediate help.

Not only is bone mass lost as a person grows older, but the main constituent of bone, calcium, is also lost. Calcium is the substance that gives bone its strength and its rigidity. The decrease in the amount of bone mass, to a point where fractures become likely, is given the name of osteoporosis. In osteoporosis, the bone is brittle. Osteoporosis, to a greater or lesser extent, affects all old people, particularly women, but in only one-quarter does a dramatic event like a fracture of wrist or hip, or the collapse of a vertebra, occur.

Osteoporosis is not a new disease. It has been found in the skeletons of prehistoric people, in the bones of primitive people and among old people in both the developed and the developing nations. Because more people in the developed nations survive the hazards of

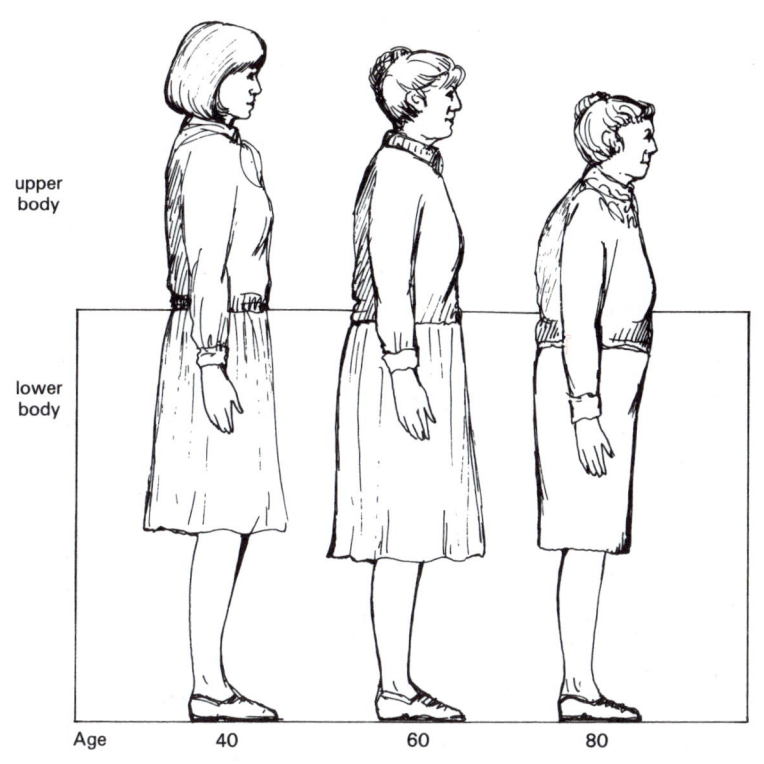

**Figure 10.1:** With increasing age, height decreases, but the decrease is of the upper spine; the length of the lower spine, the pelvis and the legs do not change

disease in childhood, more people in these countries grow old, so that osteoporosis has become more common and now constitutes a major health problem.

In three-quarters of cases, osteoporosis develops silently, but, at an unexpected time, usually following a fall or some injury, the woman's forearm or her hip fractures. Forearm fractures increase sharply among women who are aged 55 to 59, and show no consistent increase after that age. The fracture follows a fall, and falls increase in women aged 55 and over compared with younger women. A 50 year-old woman has a 1 in 6 chance of falling and fracturing her forearm (a Colles fracture), during her remaining lifetime.

As people grow older (particularly after the age of 70), their sight

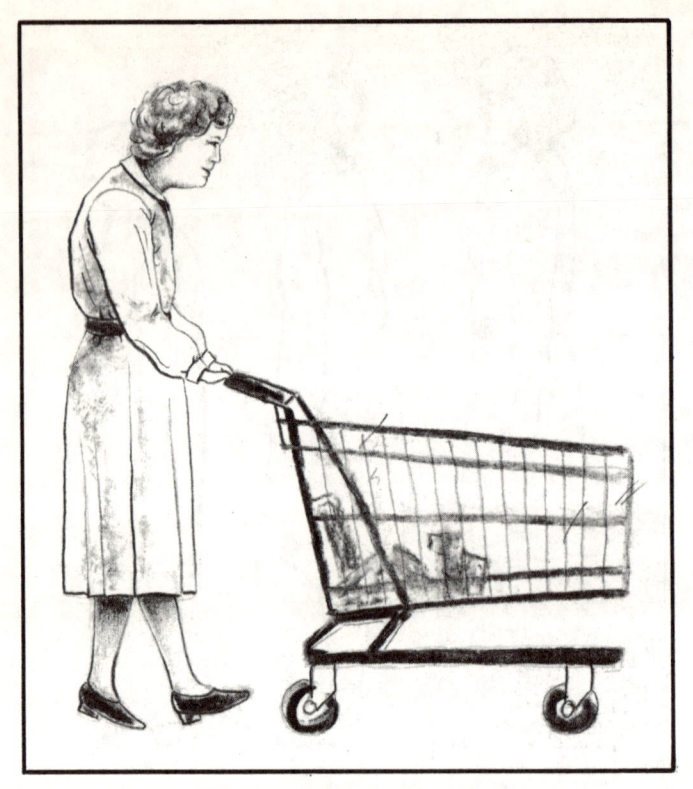

Figure 10.2: Dowager's hump

deteriorates, they become less secure on their feet and, in consequence, are more likely to sustain a fall. Older women are more frequently prescribed drugs, some of which may make them less able to maintain their balance. In the past, barbiturates caused this effect, but they are rarely prescribed today. The less dense the person's bones are, and women are more likely to have osteoporosis than men, the more likely is a woman to fracture her hip if she falls. Of course not all falls result in a hip fracture, in fact only about 7 per cent do, but the consequences can be serious. A 50 year-old white woman has been estimated to have one chance in 6 of fracturing her hip before she dies — most hip fractures occurring after the age of 70. Many of these fractures could be prevented if the woman's house had no loose rugs on the floor or other objects over which an elderly person might trip, and hand rails or other aids in strategic places that a person could hold on to to prevent her from falling. The effect of the fall on brittle bones could be reduced if the floor was carpeted.

Vertebral collapse may occur dramatically but usually the collapse slowly progresses, the woman suffering from increasing high back pain. In elderly women, the collapse of the vertebra leads to a bend in the back producing what has been called a Dowager's hump (Fig. 10.2). In some old women, several vertebrae collapse. The woman becomes shrunken, her upper body bent forward almost at a right angle to the ground, her head bent forward. In Europe from the 15th to the 18th centuries such women were often perceived to be witches and were hideously maltreated.

Osteoporosis is a disease of bone, or perhaps more accurately a degeneration of bone, which, in most cases, is due to the ageing process. To understand how the disease develops, the structure and functions of bone need to be discussed.

## BONE

In November 1974, at the Hadar in Ethiopia, Don Johanson, driving slowly in a Land-Rover through ancient lake-side deposits, looked back along the track the four-wheel drive had made. Lying on the ground he saw a fragment of fossilized bone. Searching around the fragment, Johanson and his associates eventually found other bones from the same skeleton — a lower jaw, some ribs, part of a pelvis, a thigh bone, some vertebrae and fragments of shin bone.

Careful study of the bones showed that they were of a female, about 3 feet tall, who had walked upright and had died 3 million years ago. Johanson called her Lucy. She is one of our ancestors.

Paleoanthropologists, like Don Johanson and the Leakey family, are trying to piece together the anatomy and social behaviour of mankind's ancestors from fossilized bones — all that remains of the people who lived in an area such as the Hadar and on the shores of Lake Turkana, 3 million years ago.

From this, one might infer that bone is a static, stable tissue, and that once a person is adult, bone ceases to grow and change.

Nothing could be further from the truth. Bone is almost as dynamic as skin. Bone is constantly dying and being replaced. Bone is resilient and is constantly adjusting its structure to meet new stresses. In other words, it is remodelling. Bone has a remarkable plasticity. It has these properties because of its structure and its chemical composition. Its structure comprises a covering of mem-

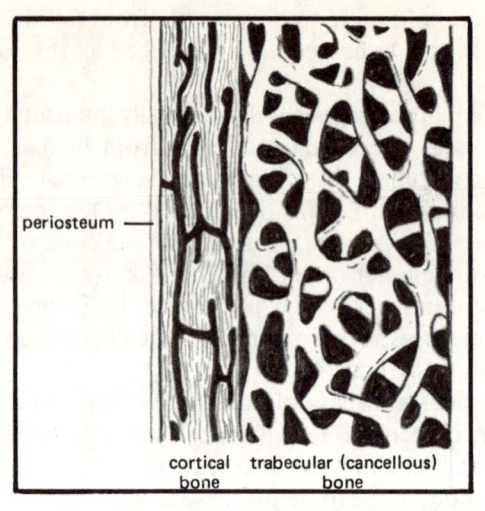

Figure 10.3: The structure of a long bone

brane, called periosteum, under which lie numerous blood vessels. Directly beneath the periosteum, there is a dense outer layer of compact bone (the cortical layer), which varies in thickness in different bones. The stronger the bone has to be, the thicker is the compact layer. For this reason, the bones of the arms and legs have thick compact layers because of the stresses they undergo, when the muscles attached to them contract. The compact bone encloses a small meshwork of spongy bone, which is made up of fine spikes of bone carefully arranged in ties and struts to give the bone stability when it is stressed by crushing or tearing. This is the spongy or trabecular layer of bone (Fig. 10.3). Inside this layer of the bones of the legs and arms is a hollow space filled with bone marrow. The vertebrae, the neck of the femur and the wrists do not have the central hollow space. Instead it is filled with trabecular bone. The vertebrae differ from the long bones in another way. Although the spinal column, which is made up of vertebrae, carries the weight of the body and needs strength, the cortical layer of each vertebral bone is rather thin, the vertebra being made up mostly of spongy bone. However, the cubical shape of each vertebra gives strength to the spine without making it impossibly heavy.

The basic substance of bone is collagen. Both the compact and the spongy layers of bone are made up of special bone cells, which secrete the protein, collagen. Collagen is relatively plastic. To give

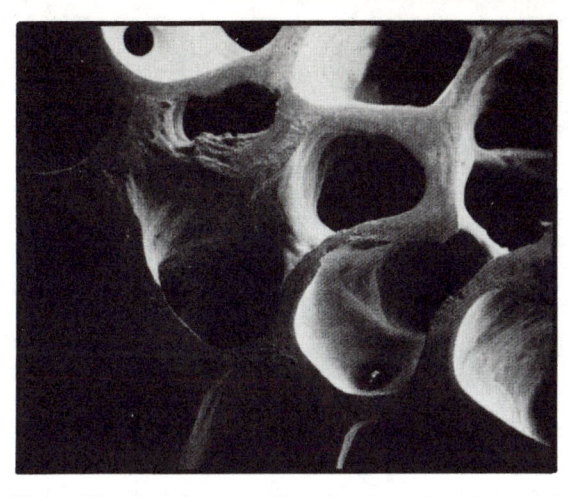

Figure 10.4: The structure of trabecular bone (courtesy of *Geriatrics* (USA))

bones rigidity and strength, it is impregnated (saturated) with lime salts, mainly calcium. If a piece of bone is placed in a weak acid solution, the calcium dissolves but the bone retains its shape, as this is dictated by the collagen framework. But now it can be twisted into knots or cut with a knife.

When a fragment of bone is examined under a microscope, its structure is shown. Compact bone consists of layers of collagen impregnated with calcium, rather like the coats of an onion. Bone cells called osteoblasts produce collagen (which is also called osteoid). These cells lie in the bone between the periosteum and the compact bone. Other bone cells called osteocytes are also present and are found between the layers of bone, looking like plum stones. They are derived from some of the osteoblasts and may contribute to the strength of the bone. Osteoblasts (in association with cells called osteoclasts) cause calcium to be deposited through the collagen to produce a 'cement'. In the spongy layer the collagen has a different distribution, being laid down in a complicated manner, which may be described as a complex honeycomb (Fig 10.4). The walls of the honeycomb are formed from collagen and impregnated with calcium, which gives the bone rigidity.

When bone dies or is changed in shape because of microscopic damage, or the need to adjust to new stresses on it, it is said to be remodelled. The remodelling of bone is going on all the time. Each

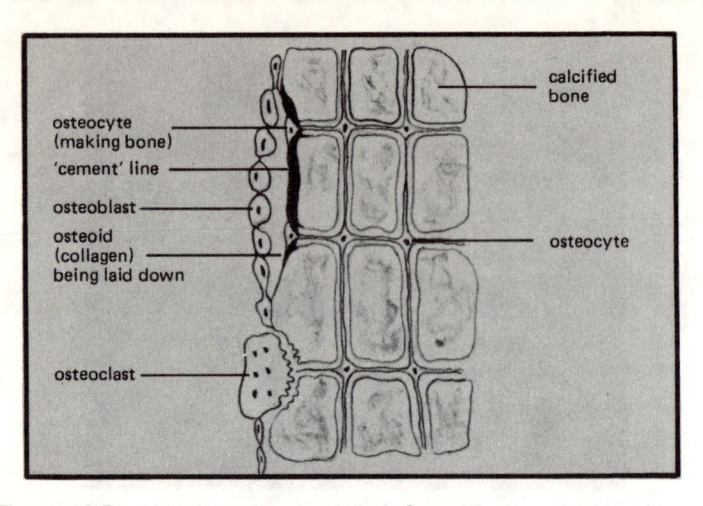

Figure 10.5: How bone is remodelled. Osteoblasts make osteoid and become enclosed in it to become osteocytes. The osteocytes together with osteoblasts (and probably osteoclasts) are involved in making calcified bone. The osteoclasts resorb calcified bone

year about 10 per cent of cortical bone and 40 per cent of trabecular bone is remodelled. Bone is first removed by the osteoclasts to a variable depth, depending on the particular bone being remodelled. The removal process (which takes about 2 weeks) ends when a line of tissue, consisting of collagen, and called the 'cement line', is laid down. On this cement line the osteoblasts lay down osteoid, which is then impregnated with calcium so that new bone is formed (Fig. 10.5). This process, which occurs in all parts of the bones, takes about 12 weeks in young people. As a person grows into late middle and old age, the process takes longer, less new osteoid being formed each day so that the process may take from 16 to 24 weeks to complete. During this time, in older people, the new osteoid formed is insufficient to replace completely the old bone that has been removed. At first, the young osteoclasts are beneficial, co-operating with osteoblasts to lay down calcium in the osteoid, which converts it into bone. Later the osteoclasts absorb bone, as just described.

This balanced process may become imbalanced in two ways. In the first way, the osteoblasts fail to make sufficient osteoid. The second way in which imbalance occurs is when the osteoblasts have a shortened life span, and die or are converted into osteoclasts before they have laid down much bone. If these changes occur, less bone is made than is removed and osteoporosis develops. As mentioned, these changes occur as a person grows older.

## CALCIUM

Calcium has a major role in mediating the many vital functions of the cells that make up a human's body. To do this effectively the level of calcium ions in the blood and in fluid that surrounds the cells of the body has to be kept in a narrow range. Calcium ions are lost constantly in the urine but the body has mechanisms to maintain the level of calcium in the blood. This is done by hormones that increase the kidney's ability to resorb calcium that would otherwise be excreted in the urine, and increase absorption of dietary calcium from the gut. However, these mechanisms need to be protected. To do this the body has a calcium 'bank' from which calcium can be withdrawn urgently when needed, and into which calcium obtained from the diet can be repaid and deposited in the calcium bank. Bone fulfils the function of the calcium bank. In fact, bone is the body's only store of calcium. As well as being essential for vital cell functions, calcium gives rigidity and strength to bone, turning soft osteoid into firm bone. If a person fails to obtain enough calcium in the diet, or needs more calcium (which occurs as women grow older) or loses too much calcium in the urine, extra calcium is removed from the bones by the osteoclasts to keep up its concentration in the blood. This in turn leads to bone remodelling.

Calcification of bone is itself a complex process and depends on a variety of mechanisms.

### How calcium is involved in bone formation

As has been mentioned, calcium (in the form of a compound called calcium hydroxyapatite) is deposited on the collagen and forms crystals, which give the bone its strength. Because bone is being remodelled constantly, calcium is released from the discarded bone and used to provide strength for the new bone. Each day about 700 g of calcium is exchanged between blood plasma and the bones. A small amount of calcium (about 150 mg) is excreted in the urine and is lost to the body, but at the same time calcium is obtained from the diet, which replaces the lost calcium.

An average European diet provides about 1100 mg of calcium each day, principally in milk and milk products such as cheese, and to a lesser extent in bread (which in England has calcium added to the flour to counteract the calcium-hoarding properties of a substance in the flour called phytate). The diet of most people in the hungry, developing world does not contain much milk. so that the amount of calcium provided is lower. In India, for example, an average of 50 mg per head per day is obtained, which is only about one-third of that provided by a European diet.

This is not such a serious situation as it might appear. Between 60 and 70 per cent of the 1100 mg of calcium in the European diet is not available for absorption. This is related in part to Western diet, which is rich in protein and high in salt, two substances that hold calcium, preventing it being absorbed. The calcium that is not absorbed is lost in the faeces. A much lower proportion of the calcium in the Indian diet is 'held' and then lost in the faeces so that relatively more is available to be absorbed. In both diets, in general, sufficient calcium is provided by food and is absorbed to replace that lost to the body.

The calcium is absorbed through the cells lining the intestine by becoming bound to protein-carriers, which transport it from the gut into the blood. Before this can happen, there must be a certain amount of vitamin $D_3$ in the body, as the protein is unable to link to calcium in the absence of this vitamin. When vitamin $D_3$ is deficient, rickets occurs in children, and the bones of adults become soft and distorted.

The absorbed calcium is transported in the blood and transferred to the bones or, if the blood level becomes too high, is excreted by the kidneys. Although the limits of the amount of calcium in the blood are strictly regulated, a constant exchange occurs from the calcium in the diet into the blood, from the blood to the bones, from the bones to the blood, from the blood to the kidneys, from the kidneys to the urine, and from the urine back into the blood or out into the lavatory pan.

The regulation of this sequence is complex, and scientists are still discovering more about how it operates. Once the calcium has been absorbed into the blood stream, the regulation of its level in the blood is controlled by two hormones. The first is a hormone produced by tiny glands found in the neck near the thyroid gland. They are called parathyroid glands and the hormone they produce is called parathyroid hormone. If the blood level of calcium falls, more parathyroid hormone is secreted. This mobilizes calcium from the bones, and by stimulating vitamin $D_3$ production in the kidneys reduces the amount lost in the urine. The second hormone involved in regulating the level of calcium in the blood is produced by the thyroid gland and is called calcitonin. Although calcitonin is known to be involved in regulating calcium in bone, how it is involved is unknown despite intense research.

These complex interactions could cause problems if anything went wrong, but, at least up to the time of the menopause, in healthy people they rarely do. This is because sufficient calcium is obtained from food to keep the blood levels normal without drawing on the calcium stores in bone. At night a slight problem arises, as most people sleep, not snack, at night. As calcium continues to be lost in the urine, its level in the blood would drop if the parathyroid hormone didn't come into play by removing a small amount of calcium from bone. But the calcium is replaced the next day from the diet.

Two other groups of hormones are also involved in regulating the loss of calcium from bone. These are the sex hormones. In women the sex hormones, oestrogen and progesterone, are produced by the ovaries. In men the sex hormone androgen is produced by the testicles.

The sex hormones protect the bones from the calcium-extracting effect of parathyroid hormone in at least two ways. First, oestrogen is involved in the synthesis of vitamin $D_3$, which in turn increases the amount of calcium absorbed from the gut. Second, oestrogen either directly or indirectly increases the secretion of calcitonin.

In most people the system works admirably. The bones, which are constantly being renewed, remain strong and rigid. The diet provides all the calcium needed to keep them strong; there is enough vitamin $D_3$ to ensure that calcium in the diet is absorbed; parathyroid hormone and calcitonin regulate the level in the body. But certain things can upset this admirable state of affairs. One is reduced mobility; another is the loss or reduction of the sex hormones.

Reduced mobility leads to a loss of calcium from bone but the effect of the loss of, or reduction in, oestrogen is much more serious.

As we discussed earlier, the level of oestrogen in the blood falls dramatically after the menopause. When this happens, first, less calcium is absorbed from the food eaten and second, the level of calcitonin may fall. The result of these two changes is that to keep up the level of calcium in the blood, the parathyroid hormone takes over to mobilize calcium from the bones, with the result that over a period of time bone tissue is resorbed. This leads to a reduction in the bone mass.

**Table 10.1:** Changes in bone mass with ageing

---

Bone loss occurs when resorption exceeds formation

*Trabecular bone* (vertebrae, neck femur, lower end radius)
Gain till age 25–30
Loss from age 40–45 onwards:
    40–50   0.3–1.0% per annum
    50–60   3.0–5.0% per annum in women
    60+     0.3–1.0% per annum

*Cortical bone* (long bones of arms and legs)
Gain till age 30
Loss from age 40–45 onwards — ? a steady loss at 0.5–1.0% per annum

---

## CHANGES IN BONE MASS WITH AGEING

A person's bone mass increases up to the age of about 30, when it reaches its 'peak' (Table 10.1). At this age, the amount of bone a person has depends in part on genetic inheritance ('choosing the right parents'), and in part good nutrition during childhood and young adult life. Of course, nobody can choose their parents, but if there is a family history of osteoporosis, the woman should be particularly aware of the need to increase the amount of calcium she obtains each day to at least 800 mg, preferably from food, (see Table 4.2 page 37), and to take regular exercise. These measures should start at the age of 12. Good nutrition includes more than maintaining a high calcium intake each day. It implies that the person eats a diet which is rich in complex carbohydrates, vitamins and fibre (cereals, vegetables, legumes and fruit); has about 10 per cent of protein; and is relatively low in saturated fats.

From about the age of 30 (perhaps earlier), the bone mass remains unaltered (or there is a small loss not exceeding 0.5 per cent a year), until the woman reaches the menopause when the loss of bone increases to an average of 2 to 3 per cent a year for about 10 years, although the loss in a few women is higher, up to 8 per cent being lost each year. After this time, for some unknown reason, the bone loss decreases to about 0.5 per cent a year.

Over an average lifetime of 75 years, a woman may lose about 25 to 35 per cent of her cortical bone, which is the major component of the bones of the arms and legs. Over the same lifetime, a woman may lose 40 to 50 per cent of her spongy (trabecular) bone. Because men produce the male sex hormone androgen into old age, they are luckier, losing only about two-thirds of women's bone loss.

Bone loss does not occur at a regular rate and, as well, the proportion of bone lost varies between individuals. The effect of the bone loss also varies — the more bone originally, the fewer will be the clinical effects of osteoporosis.

These two factors show that the likelihood of a woman developing osteoporosis depends, first, on the amount of bone she has (her peak bone mass), and, second, the rate at which she loses bone after the menopause. If in the years before the menopause she ceases to menstruate for one year or more (for example if she has anorexia nervosa, or is a long-distance runner), or if she is required to take corticosteroid drugs for long periods, she will lose bone more rapidly than usual and may develop osteoporosis at an earlier age.

There is some controversy about the rate of bone loss from trabecular and from cortical bone. This is because different methods of estimating bone loss give different results.

The consensus is that trabecular bone begins to be lost from about the age of 35. The loss is mainly from the vertebrae, the wrists and the lower jaw. At first the rate of loss is slow, averaging 0.5 per cent of trabecular bone mass each year. As mentioned, once a woman reaches the menopause, the rate of trabecular bone loss increases to between 3 and 5 per cent a year. This rate of bone loss persists for 5 to 10 years after which the rate slows to between 0.5 and 1 per cent.

Cortical bone loss starts about a decade later than trabecular bone loss, at the age of 45 in both sexes. The initial rate of loss is 0.3 to 0.5 per cent each year. In women the rate of loss increases to 2 to 3 per cent in the 5 to 10 years after the menopause, and then the rate decreases to 0.3 to 0.5 per cent a year.

Not all women lose bone at the same rate. A Swiss study of 35 women followed for 3 years after their menopause showed that half of them did not lose bone; a quarter lost between 1 and 2 per cent of their bone mass, and a quarter lost larger amounts (up to 14 per cent) of their bone mass. The women who lost bone had phases when relatively little bone was lost, followed by phases of increased bone loss.

The reasons for the different rates of bone loss are not clear, but studies show that women who are thin, who smoke, who consume alcohol heavily, who are prescribed certain drugs and whose calcium intake from food is low, may lose bone at a greater rate and may be more likely to develop the clinical signs of osteoporosis.

Men have a larger bone mass and do not experience the hormonal changes of the menopause. Consequently they do not have the increased rate of bone loss until the age of 70. After the age of 70 the pattern of bone loss changes. Men and women now lose bone at an equal rate.

When the density of the bone falls below a critical level, fractures occur. The vertebrae are affected particularly and 'wedge' fractures become common. The collapse of the vertebra leads to the 'Dowager's hump' (See Fig. 10.3). Fracture of the hip is increasingly common with ageing and because women have lost more bone before the age of 70 than men, twice as many elderly women fracture their hips compared with men.

## WHAT LEADS TO OSTEOPOROSIS?

At present the reason why older people, especially women, develop osteoporosis is also not clear. Several factors have been suggested. These include:

- reduced levels of sex hormones
- taking less exercise
- reduced calcium intake or absorption
- smoking
- ? increased tea or coffee consumption (by increasing calcium loss in the urine)
- ? increased alcohol consumption.

*Reduced levels of sex hormones*  During the reproductive years, at least until the menopause, oestrogen produced by the woman's ovaries prevents bone loss. (In men, the male hormone androgen has the same effect.) The effect of oestrogen is indirect because no 'receptors' for oestrogen have been found in bone. (There may be receptors on the osteoblasts.) This means that oestrogen acts by suppressing the activity of bone-resorbing hormones, such as the parathyroid gland hormone; or by increasing the effect of calcitonin, or by increasing the quantity of calcium absorbed from the gut; or by reducing the loss of calcium in the urine. The decline in the level of oestrogen circulating in the blood, which occurs at and after the menopause, seems to be the major factor leading to osteoporosis in women.

*Reduced mobility*  Middle-aged people, especially women, tend to take less exercise than when they were younger and this is one of the factors that over the years may lead to osteoporosis, as exercise is known to increase the amount of calcium in the bones. The loss of bone in middle-aged women may be greater than that of middle aged men, because women lack androgen — the male sex hormone — which protects against bone loss. Androgen secretion is increased by exercise and this may be one way in which exercise helps to prevent osteoporosis.

*Reduced calcium intake and absorption*  The strength and rigidity of bone is dependent on calcium salts being deposited on the meshwork of collagen that makes up bone. As people grow older, they absorb less dietary calcium from their gut; and women who have osteoporosis tend to absorb less than other women of a similar age. As was discussed earlier, a negative calcium balance leads to osteoporosis. The additional loss of calcium is due, in part, to the lack of circulating oestrogen which permits an increasing urinary loss of oestrogen and, in part, to calcium loss in the faeces (motions).

A further factor is that postmenopausal women need to absorb twice as much calcium to prevent deficiency, compared with younger women or men. The reason for this is complex and may be related to the reduction in oestrogen circulating in a woman's body after the menopause.

To remain in calcium balance, a woman who is postmenopausal should take 1500 mg of calcium a day in her food or as a calcium supplement.

With these facts known, it is unfortunate that many menopausal women reduce their intake of diary foods (milk and cheese).

*Smoking*  There is evidence that women who smoke have an earlier menopause and that osteoporosis occurs earlier and is more severe if the woman smokes. This is because smoking may damage the ovaries and in some way increases the metabolism of the sex hormones by the liver so that a lower level of circulating oestrogen is available to prevent bone loss.

*Increased ingestion of caffeine and alcohol*  Some studies suggest that an increased ingestion of caffeine is a factor in the development of osteoporosis by increasing the loss of calcium in the urine. Middle-aged women tend to drink more tea and coffee than younger women, and a few drink more alcohol. However, it has not been proved that the increased caffeine and alcohol increase the likelihood of developing osteoporosis.

## THE SYMPTOMS OF OSTEOPOROSIS

In itself, bone loss in most women is symptomless, but if an accident occurs, such as a fall, the weakened bone may break or collapse. Older people are more likely to experience a fall, and the longer the person lives, the greater is the chance that she or he will have a fall. This is because older people are more likely to have a dizzy episode. Their sight is less acute. They may suddenly lose their balance. They may be taking antidepressant medication, which may cause a sudden fall in blood pressure, or they may be taking drugs to treat their high blood pressure. The effects of the fall vary. Whether the fall will cause a bone fracture depends on how much bone mass the person has and on the quality of the bone. This can be summarized as:

$$\frac{\text{liability to fall} \times \text{length of life}}{\text{bone mass} \times \text{bone quality}}$$

Within a community, the frequency of bone fractures amongst older women gives some indication of the extent of the problem of osteoporosis in that community.

In the USA, osteoporosis affects over 10 million of the 30 million women who are aged more than 50, and is responsible for over one million fractures each year: 700 000 being vertebral fractures and 200 000 of them being hip fractures. The direct and indirect costs of caring for osteoporosis sufferers in the USA have been estimated at over $US10 billion. In Britain, over 50 000 women sustain a hip fracture each year. The cost of all osteoporotic fractures in Britain was estimated in 1988 to be £500 million, which was three times more than the costs of hospital treatment of hip fractures alone. In Australia, about 10 000 older women sustain a hip fracture each year at a cost to the community of over $A200 million.

In all of these countries, the number of people over the age of 60 is increasing at about 2 per cent a year, and a person aged 60 has a life expectancy of between 15 and 25 years. This means that in the next decades more people are likely to experience a fall and, unless the prevalence of osteoporosis can be reduced, the costs of treating people will double or treble in the next 20 years.

As was noted in the American studies, the bones that make up the spinal column, the vertebrae, are most frequently affected. In most women over the age of 50, vertebral bones become slowly, insidiously brittle (Fig. 10.6). Over this period, it is likely that tiny

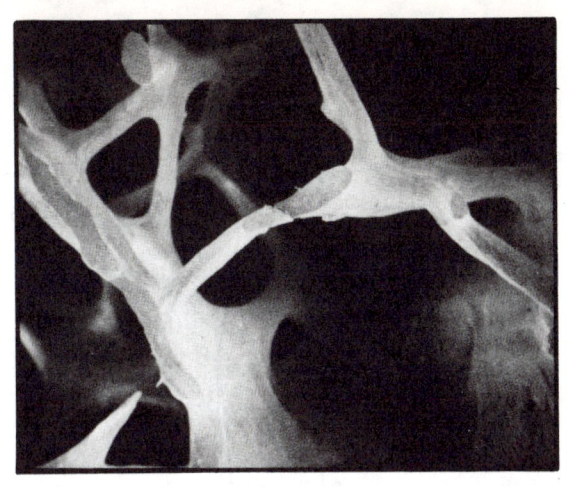

Figure 10.6: The structure of osteoporotic bone — compare with Figure 10.4 (courtesy of *Geriatrics* (USA))

fractures occur in some of the slender ties and struts that make up spongy bone. For many years this process is without symptoms, but the woman gradually loses height and may develop a 'Dowager's hump'. The loss in height may be small, but one woman in eight loses 20 per cent of her height between the age of 50 and 70 (Fig 10.7). In a few women the bone loss from the vertebrae leads to a sudden complete collapse of a vertebra — a compression fracture. This is accompanied by severe back pain. The compression fracture may be initiated by a routine activity such as bending, rising from a chair or bed or lifting an object.

But in most women, the vertebral compression occurs without symptoms and leads to a reduction in the woman's height. Sometimes the woman has intermittent pain from spasms of the back muscles, which now have to take a greater share in supporting the upper part of the body. In the most severe cases the woman's back becomes bent and she develops a 'witch like' posture. This occurs in about three women in every hundred between the age of 40 and 60 and in seven women in every hundred over the age of 60.

Two other fractures occur increasingly with age and both are more common in women than in men (at least before the age of 80). Studies in Sweden in the 1960s and in the USA in the 1980s show

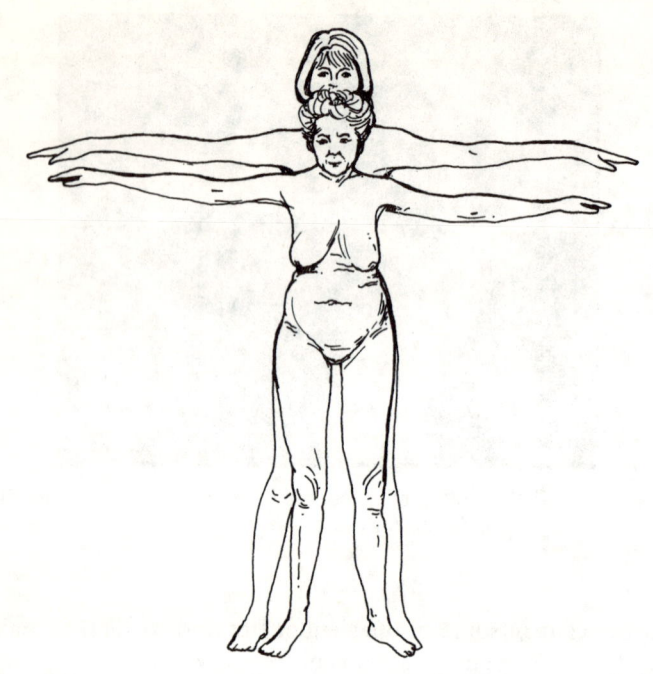

**Figure 10.7:** When this woman was aged 40 her height was 165 cm (5 ft 6 ins). At age 80, her height is 156 cm (5 ft 2½ ins).

that fractures of the lower end of the forearm (Colles fracture) and the hip increase as a person ages (Figure 10.8). Most hip fractures occur after the age of 70 in both sexes. Over the age of 75, one woman in every three and one of every six men will sustain a hip fracture. Hip fractures are disabling, costly to treat and often life threatening. In 1980, in the USA, of the 230 000 elderly people who had a hip fracture one in ten died within six months and between a quarter and a half were never able to walk or to function as well. Many of these elderly people had to remain in nursing homes permanently.

The incidence of hip fractures also has been increasing in Britain in the past decade, as studies from Nottingham show. The studies confirm that men and women over the age of 65 are at the greatest risk, and that in each age group after 65 years, women are at greater risk than men. About 50 000 people in Britain fracture a hip each year.

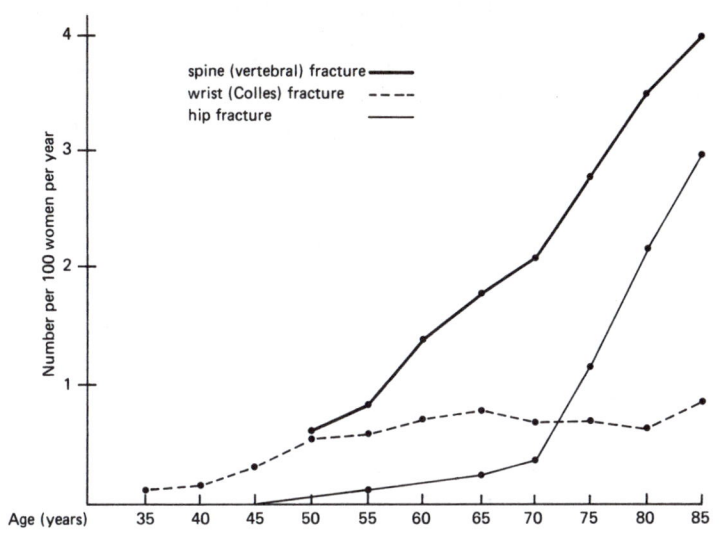

Figure 10.8: Incidence (per 100 women per year in each age group) of three common fractures

Taken together, collapse of a vertebra or the fracture of the forearm or the hip affect about one woman in four over the age of 60. Although all women lose bone, only 25 per cent develop symptomatic osteoporosis.

In any one year, about 2 per cent of women between the age of 45 and 64 years and 3 per cent of women aged 65 or older will break a bone, usually a bone in the forearm or, less commonly, one of her thigh bones (the neck of the femur), following a fall. As a 65 year-old woman has a life expectancy of about 19 years, she has a 15 per cent chance, particularly as she grows older, of fracturing the neck of her femur because of osteoporosis.

Not only do brittle bones lead to an increase in fractures, new evidence suggests that women who have osteoporosis have a higher chance of dying from stroke compared with women who do not have osteoporosis. The reason is not clear but may be connected with the belief that the women who have brittle bones are less healthy than other women, and take less exercise: conditions which may be involved in the development of osteoporosis.

## PREVENTING OSTEOPOROSIS

*Prevention is crucial as few treatments significantly increase bone mass once it is lost and when they do, they predominantly affect trabecular (spongy) bone mass, sometimes at the expense of cortical (the solid) bone mass.*

C. N. de Deuxchaisnes, 1983

Despite the lack of scientific evidence that osteoporosis can be prevented, the interplay of various factors discussed provides a rational basis for treatment that may delay, or prevent, osteoporosis (Table 10.2). It is one that every woman can follow.

**Table 10.2:** Possible ways to prevent or delay osteoporosis

* Take ½ to 1 hour of exercise three times a week
* Take 1.5 g of calcium each day as dairy products or a calcium tablet
* Reduce or stop cigarette smoking
* Limit the amount of alcohol you take
* Discuss with a doctor whether or not to take small daily doses of oestrogens (and progestogens) at least for the first 5 to 10 years after your menopause
* Avoid taking barbiturates as they seem to increase the fracture rate

### Calcium intake

As the bones increase in density from the age of 12 to about the age of 30, this is a period during which calcium intake should be kept high. Young people, especially women, should make sure that they obtain at least 800 mg of calcium in their daily diet. This amount can be obtained from about 750 ml of milk (whole or skimmed) or 90 g of cheese (Table 10.3).

Women from about the age of 35 should make sure that they increase their calcium intake in an effort to counteract the osteoporotic process. From the time of the menopause an increased calcium intake is probably even more important. Peri- and postmenopausal women should ingest at least 1500 mg of calcium a day.

Skimmed milk provides 1 mg of calcium per millilitre and 90 g of cheese contains around 800 mg of calcium. If a woman prefers not to eat dairy products, she can buy calcium supplements. Argument,

Table 10.3: Calcium content of typical average servings of common foods

| Food | Calcium (mg) | Serving size |
|---|---|---|
| Milk (whole or skimmed) | 280 | 250 mL |
| Yoghurt | 310 | 200 g |
| Swiss cheese | 285 | 30 g |
| Cheddar cheese | 260 | 30 g |
| Processed cheese | 205 | 30 g |
| Cottage cheese | 190 | 200 g |
| Canned salmon | 110 | ¼ cup |
| Broccoli | 60 | 60 g |
| Orange | 60 | 150 g |
| Fish | 50 | 100 g |
| Baked beans | 40 | 100 g |
| Egg | 30 | 55 g |
| Carrots | 30 | 90 g |
| French beans | 30 | 60 g |
| Bran flakes | 20 | 30 g |
| Steak | 20 | 100 g |
| Bread (slice) | 10 | 25 g |
| Potato | 10 | (large) |

*Source:* Dairy Corporation (NSW).

among specialist physicians, continues about which is the most effective calcium preparation. But it is agreed that at least some calcium should be taken in the evening, as the greatest loss of calcium from bone occurs during sleep.

Controversy and debate, often heated and emotional, continues between groups of doctors who are involved in osteoporosis research, whether calcium has any protective value in preventing osteoporosis.

Three investigations made in the USA in the past 12 years have suggested that calcium in a dose of about 1.5 g daily (1 g of which is preferably taken at night), from the time of the menopause helps to prevent bone loss and reduce the risk of hip fracture later in life. Three other equally reliable studies show that additional calcium after the menopause has no effect on reducing bone loss or on preventing fractures. The reason for the lack of agreement has now been found. It is this. Women who have a low daily intake of calcium (less than 500 mg a day) can reduce their bone loss by increasing their calcium intake to over 1000 mg a day, but women whose calcium intake is 800 mg a day or more, will not reduce their risk of developing osteoporosis by taking calcium supplements.

### Sex hormones, particularly oestrogen

At least there is agreement about oestrogen. All doctors who treat menopausal women agree that daily doses of oestrogen will reduce bone loss from the vertebrae and probably the long bones of women who have passed the menopause. For example, a group of doctors in California, led by Dr Ettinger, found that the height of postmenopausal women who took small doses of oestrogen each day did not decrease and their risk of developing a fracture of a vertebra was half that of women who did not take oestrogen. The risk of a wrist fracture was halved and that of a hip fracture reduced two and a half times.

The researchers made another interesting observation. If oestrogen (in a dose of 0.01 mg of ethinyl oestradiol or equivalent) was given together with calcium, this lower dose was effective in preventing significant bone loss from the spine and the long bones of the body. Recently, some doubt has been expressed that the combination of oestrogen and calcium has any benefit over that of oestrogen alone.

Research since 1980 has shown that the dose of oestrogen needed to prevent bone loss is critical. A daily dose of Premarin or Ogen of 0.625 mg, or an equivalent dose of the other oestrogens with the exception of ethinyl oestradiol which requires at least 20 mg (see Table 8.2 p. 68), will protect the woman against bone loss. As was noted on page 69, women who have not had a hysterectomy, and who choose to take oestrogen require to take a progestogen for 12 days each month, to protect the uterus from undue stimulation by oestrogen.

Interestingly, there is some evidence that progestogen also helps to prevent bone loss and may produce bone formation. Studies have shown that a progestogen given each day will prevent bone loss — but not as effectively as oestrogen. A possible problem of progestogen treatment is that some women develop premenstrual tension-like symptoms (for example, irritability and tender breasts).

A new hormone, Livial, is also effective in preventing bone loss and appears to increase bone density. This hormone has been referred to on page 74 and may be preferred to oestrogen by some women.

It is not clear how long a woman should take hormone replacement treatment to prevent bone loss and the development of osteoporosis. As bone loss is greatest for the 5 to 10 years after the menopause, oestrogen should be taken for this time. But oestrogen has other benefits, particularly in reducing the chance of heart attack, which suggests that oestrogen should be continued for longer than 10 years.

## Hormone replacement treatment or routine bone density scanning?

Only a few women, less than 15 per cent of all women aged 50–59, currently agree to take HRT for prolonged periods of time. For this reason the question has to be asked: Is it economically sensible for all post-menopausal women to take oestrogen for 10 years or longer? A mathematical model made in Britain has shown that oestrogen, taken in this way, will reduce the risk of hip fracture by 40 per cent. However, many women have to be convinced of the benefit of continuing to take hormone replacement treatment for long periods of time.

For women who choose not to take HRT, is there any way of identifying the women most at risk of developing osteoporosis? The answer is that the density of the bones can be tested. If this were done, it is likely, mathematically at least, that the same reduction in osteoporosis would occur if only those women who had a low bone density took oestrogen. However, the finding that the bones are less dense only shows that the woman is *more likely* to sustain a fracture in later life, it does not say that she *will* fracture a bone.

Machines are available which measure the mineral density of the cortical bones in the forearm or hip or the trabecular bone in the spine. Many investigators have shown that for an accurate prediction about the likelihood of osteoporosis occurring in the menopausal years, measurements should be made of both the trabecular bones in the spine and the cortical bones in the forearm or hip. A new machine using a very low dose of X-rays is available, which measures the bone density in both the spine and that of the hip-bone or forearm with a high degree of accuracy and gives the result quickly using a computer print out. This is a 'dual energy X-ray absorptiometry' (DEXA) machine.

There is another item in assessing the risk of a woman developing osteoporosis. This is the *rate* of bone loss after the menopause. For example, a woman who has a high bone density at the menopause and a rapid rate of bone loss (say 5 to 7 per cent per year) will be as likely to develop osteoporosis as a woman who has a low bone density at the menopause but a low rate of bone loss (less than 2 per cent per year).

There are two ways in which the rate of bone loss can be estimated. The first is to perform bone density scanning every two years or so, to find out the rate of bone loss. The second, which some scientists believe is as accurate and more convenient, is to measure the bone mineral density once at the time of the menopause and, at the same time, to measure certain biochemical substances in the blood and urine (osteocalcin, alkaline phosphàtase and hydroxyproline). The scientists claim that their method will give as accurate a prediction of the rate of bone loss (at least in the next 5 years) and the risk that the woman will develop osteoporosis as frequent bone mineral density measurements; and will predict which women are fast bone losers and which are slow bone losers.

Whichever method is chosen, three groups of women can be identified: (1) women who have a low mineral bone density and a rapid or intermediate rate of bone loss; (2) women who have an intermediate or high bone mineral density and a high or intermediate rate of bone loss, and (3) women who have a high bone density and a low rate of bone loss. Women in the first group would be wise to take HRT (or one of the other drugs which delay the loss of bone, page 117) to prevent osteoporosis. Women in the second group might choose to avoid HRT and take the other measures which delay the onset of osteoporosis (see p. 112). These women should have their bone mineral density rechecked after 2 to 3 years.

Women in the third group would not need to take HRT for the prevention of osteoporosis, although it would be valuable treatment to reduce the risk of coronary heart disease.

Because of the effectiveness of hormone replacement treatment in preventing osteoporosis in all menopausal women, it is questionable if bone density measurements are worth making on all postmenopausal women.

This opinion has been supported by several consensus conferences in which the experts agreed that *routine* bone mineral density screening is neither cost effective nor does it benefit the individual woman, unless she chooses not to take hormone replacement treatment, or ceases to take it after the menopausal symptoms have ceased.

### Exercise

The amount of exercise taken daily should be increased. The exercise need not be strenuous, but should be sufficient to put 'stress' on the spine and the legs. A brisk walk or rather energetic gardening are as beneficial as any other kind of exercise. Exercise should be taken for half to one hour three times a week. Evidence from the USA and from Australia shows that this amount of exercise, over a period of a year, increased the bone mass (determined by measuring the total amount of calcium in the body) of menopausal women by 2.5 per cent, while a 'control group' of similar age, eating habits and socioeconomic status, who were sedentary, had lost 2.5 per cent of their total bone mass by the end of the year.

### Other treatments for preventing osteoporosis

Some women either cannot or do not want to take hormones to prevent osteoporosis. If this is their choice, other treatments are possible, although they are more expensive.

One of these treatment is for the woman to take a drug called calcitonin, although the treatment is controversial. Calcitonin prevents bone loss from the vertebral skeleton but does not prevent bone loss from the long bones of the arms and legs. One form of calcitonin is given by sniffing it (salmon calcitonin), and another form is given by injection (carbo calcitonin). Calcitonin appears to be as effective in preventing bone loss in the spine as oestrogen but is more expensive.

Fluoride has been tried and certainly thickens the compact outer layer of long bones, which may add to its strength. Fluoride also thickens the struts and ties of spongy bone, but paradoxically, this may make the bone less able to resist twisting stresses and more likely to fracture. The authors of two recent studies say that fluoride should not be used to prevent or to treat established osteoporosis, as it is ineffective.

Recently a new method of preventing osteoporosis has been suggested. This is for the woman to take a new drug, etidronate, which will be discussed later in this chapter.

Androgens or anabolic testosterone have been suggested as an alternative to oestrogen treatment. The argument is that men, who secrete testosterone, lose bone more slowly than women, and that therefore androgens protect against bone loss. However, careful investigations show that androgens are less effective than oestrogens in *preventing* bone loss but may be useful in *treating* osteoporosis.

## THE TREATMENT OF ESTABLISHED, DEFORMING OSTEOPOROSIS

Many women do not seek help to prevent the development of osteoporosis, many others are unaware of treatment which would prevent this disabling disease. As mentioned earlier, fewer than 15 per cent of women in their early post menopausal years take hormone replacement treatment regularly. For these reasons osteoporosis continues to cause health problems for many elderly women. Because of this, the treatment of established osteoporosis requires to be discussed.

It must first be said that it is much more difficult to treat established osteoporosis than to prevent this disabling disorder. Several treatments have been advocated for established osteoporosis, which offer a choice to women who have deforming osteoporosis. The treatments are: (1) Sex hormone treatments: oestrogen (HRT), and Livial. (2) Etidronate (Didronel). (3) Calcitonin and (4) Nandrolone decanoate (Deca Durabolin).

### Sex hormone treatment

HRT to treat *established* osteoporosis by preventing further bone resorption has been reported as beneficial by some scientists and as of no value by others. On balance it seems that women treated with HRT over a period of 2 years increase their bone mineral density in the lumbar spine by up to 6 per cent, and in the femoral neck by up to 3 per cent. As well, the women studied had a slightly decreased vertebral fracture rate. The dose of oestrogen chosen is that mentioned when the prevention of osteoporosis was discussed. If the woman is over 60 years of age and has not been taking oestrogenic hormones, she would be sensible to start with a very small dose of oestrogen and build up the dose slowly to reduce the chance of side effects of the treatment. One of the side effects is a return of menstrual bleeding in women who have not had a hysterectomy. The evidence from several countries is that about two-thirds of women have not had the operation by the age of 55. Of course, these women will need to take a progestogen for 12 days a month, to protect their endometrium against the chance of uterine cancer, and on ceasing each progestogen course they will usually have a 'period'. Some women, whether they have had a hysterectomy or not, who take HRT for established osteoporosis develop breast tenderness and sometimes breast pain.

The return of menstrual bleeding seems to be the most annoying side effect for many women. Over 70 per cent of English and Dutch post menopausal women questioned stated that they objected to restarting their 'periods' after the menopause. However it is believed that many women, under the age of 70, will accept the 'periods,' which are usually light, if explanation and counselling are provided.

Two other hormonal regimens, currently under investigation, are to prescribe continuous combined oestrogen and progestogen or for the woman to choose the new hormone, Livial. If either of these treatments are chosen, the woman may expect to have irregular, unpredictable bleeds in the first 3 or 4 months but after this she may expect few or no withdrawal bleeds. Both treatments provide as much protection from endometrial stimulation as do the usual regimens of HRT. Both protect against further bone loss, and Livial, after a few months use, actually increases bone formation.

## Etidronate

Etidronate is a drug which inhibits the reabsorption of bone by the osteoclasts, allowing the osteoblasts to make new bone. Because of this effect the drug should be of value in treating established osteoporosis. Studies in the USA and Sweden show that etidronate (Didronel), in a dose of 400 mg a day for 14 days every 3 months increases bone mass by 2 to 3 per cent each year and reduces the number of vertebral fractures by 50 per cent. During the 13 weeks interval between treatments, the woman is given additional calcium. The concept behind intermittent treatment is that the osteoblasts and osteoclasts communicate with each other. When bone resorption is suppressed, bone formation is also reduced, but only after an interval of two or three months. During the interval osteoblasts lay down new bone. The beneficial effect on bone continues for at least 2 years. Some concern has been expressed by the Food and Drug Administration of the USA that in the third year of etidronate use, vertebral fractures may *increase*. Until this matter is resolved, etidronate is only available for research purposes.

Unfortunately, etidronate has some adverse effects: between 5 and 10 per cent of women are nauseated or have diarrhoea, but the symptoms are usually mild.

## Calcitonin

Initial research using injections of salmon calcitonin suggested that the calcitonin prevented the progressive loss of bone mass, at least for the first 2 or 3 years of use. More recent studies using calcitonin have shown that although it reduces further bone loss in the vertebrae and in the femur, it does not reduce the rate of new fractures of the vertebral bone in women who have established osteoporosis, and its use should be confined to research programmes.

## Nandrolone decanoate

The steroid hormone, nandrolone decanoate (Deca-Durabolin), in a dose of 50 mg given into a muscle every 3 to 4 weeks, has been shown to increase bone mass by inhibiting bone resorption and by stimulating bone formation. It is the only treatment which has this combined effect. Most of the benefit occurs in the first year of having the injections (but may continue as long as the woman continues to have the injections).

A problem associated with the use of nandrolone decanoate is that one-third of women report that their voice becomes hoarse after 6 months of treatment, and about one woman in twenty finds that her body hair increases in amount.

## Fluoride

Fluoride increases trabecular but not cortical bone mass, and may even reduce the latter, so that calcium has to be given as well to try to prevent this happening. Unfortunately, in spite of initial promise, fluoride treatment does not appear to reduce the rate of vertebral fractures, which are the most common fractures in postmenopausal women. As well, about a quarter of women taking fluoride develop gastrointestinal upsets, joint and bone pain, and one-third fail to respond to fluoride treatment. Recent studies indicate that fluoride should no longer be used to treat established osteoporosis.

## Calcitriol (vitamin $D_3$)

Once the favoured treatment of osteoporosis, large doses of vitamin D have not been found to improve bone mass when compared with a placebo, except in women whose diet is deficient in vitamin D. This is uncommon in Western countries, but may occur in some elderly women whose diet is poor.

Recently the use of calcitriol, the active form of vitamin D has been used to treat osteoporosis. Calcitriol increases the absorption of calcium from the gut and induces osteoblast cells to produce bone. Some studies show that calcitriol is useful; others find no benefit.

The largest study conducted in New Zealand suggests that calcitriol, if taken daily for 2 years or more, reduces new fractures in the spine, and may increase the density of the vertebrae. It has no effect on the long bones. If the early promise is confirmed, calcitriol may be another treatment for osteoporosis.

## Calcium

It may seem strange to leave calcium to the end of this section, as calcium is recommended to be taken by young women to increase their 'bone bank'. The reason is that once the person's 'bone bank' ceases to grow at about the age of 40, calcium has little effect on bone provided that the diet provides an adequate amount.

A few scientists still believe that calcium supplements given will prevent further bone fractures in established osteoporosis, but most find that calcium is of no benefit, unless the woman's diet is very low in calcium-containing foods. Women who have a low daily intake of calcium (less than 500 mg a day), may reduce their bone loss by increasing their calcium intake to over 1000 mg a day, but women whose calcium intake is 800 mg a day or more, derive no benefit from calcium.

## The future

Research is progressing into this important area and it is hoped that in the near future an effective treatment for osteoporosis, which has few or no side effects, will have been found. The importance of preventing this crippling disease remains paramount.

# 11
# THE MIDDLE YEARS AND THE BODY SYSTEMS

As a woman passes through her middle years, and particularly after she has passed her menopause, she becomes more liable to develop certain medical conditions which may affect her enjoyment of life. During these years she is more likely to develop heart and circulatory problems, particularly coronary heart disease; she may find that she is less well able to control her urine and may 'wet' herself from time to time; she may develop a 'prolapse' of her genital organs; she may start bleeding from her vagina and she has an increasing risk of developing breast cancer.

These are the issues which will be discussed in this chapter.

## HEART AND CIRCULATORY PROBLEMS

Studies of the incidence of coronary heart disease show that at all ages women are less likely to have a heart attack than are men. As a woman grows older the difference diminishes, but it persists throughout life. For example, only 2 women aged 40 to 49 in every 1000 and 6 women aged 50 to 59 in every 1000 are likely to suffer a heart attack each year compared with six times as many men in the 40–49 age group and four times as many men in the age group 50–59. Of the women who have a heart attack only 1 in 7 aged 40–49 and 1 in 5 aged 50–59 will die as a result of the heart attack, whilst 1 man in 5 in the age group 40–49 and 1 man in 3 in the 50–59 age group is likely to die after a heart attack.

As people grow older, the difference between men and women both in the frequency of heart attack and of death following a heart attack, diminishes further and by the age of 60 only twice as many men as women will have a heart attack (Fig. 11.1).

Coronary heart disease is a common reason for a person dying

CHD MORTALITY (PER 100,000)

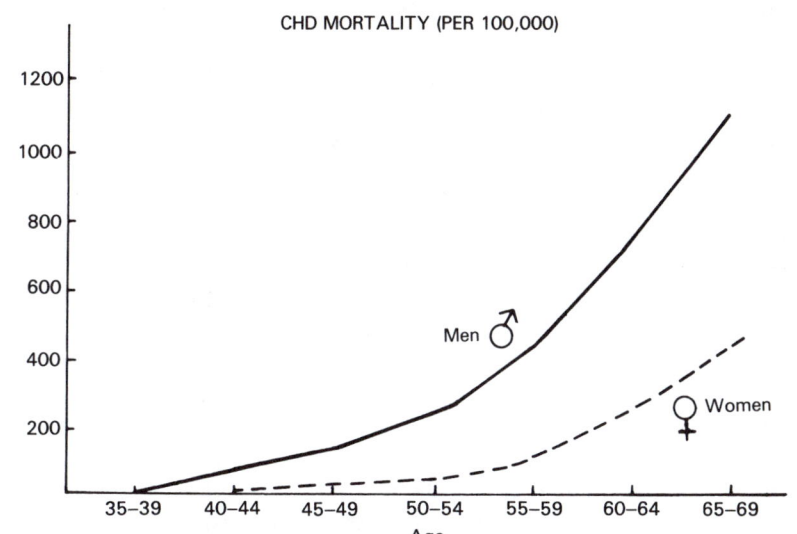

Figure 11.1: Deaths from coronary heart disease per 100 000 of the population (England and Wales 1987-89)

prematurely, often in the prime of life. In consequence, a great deal of research has been made to try and find out what are the 'risk factors' for the disease. Risk factors are usually considered to be lifestyle behaviours which increase the chance that the individual will have a heart attack, and which, if corrected, reduce that chance.

Scientists have found that these following factors increase the risk of having a heart attack:

- the amount of fat (particularly saturated fat) in the diet;
- cigarette smoking;
- lack of exercise;
- high blood pressure;
- obesity (particularly in women);
- diabetes.

Women and men tend to eat the same kind of food; as many women as men have high blood pressure and diabetes so that these cannot be the reason that fewer women than men have coronary heart disease. In past years more men than women smoked and this might be the reason, but the difference is diminishing as more women are now smoking tobacco.

This seems to suggest that the main reason why fewer women than men suffer a heart attack (at least in the years up to the woman's menopause), is because of her sex — a woman's ovaries produce oestrogen. The protective effect of oestrogen is demonstrated by the observation that if a woman has had a hysterectomy and her ovaries removed in her thirties, she has twice the chance of having a heart attack compared with a woman who has not had the operation. The importance of this observation will be discussed later.

Obesity is a particular risk factor for a middle-aged woman, particularly if the obesity is 'abdominal obesity', that is if the circumference of her waist exceeds the circumference of her hips. The greater the waist measurement is, compared with the hip measurement, the greater is the risk that the woman will have a heart attack. Women who are fat, that is their Body Mass Index is 30 or more, have twice the risk of having a heart attack compared with women whose weight is in the normal range (BMI 20–24.9). Fig. 11.2.

Fat in the diet needs further consideration as at present there is much discussion by doctors and by the public about the role of fat in the diet as a cause of heart disease. There is now strong evidence that the dietary fat is an important risk factor for coronary heart disease.

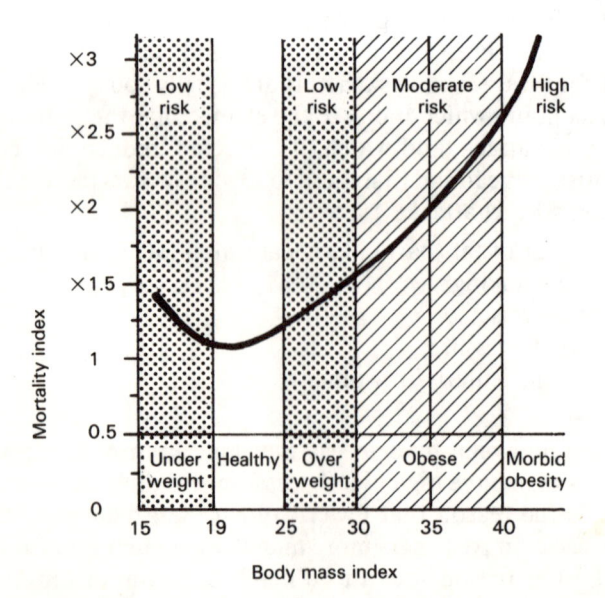

Figure 11.2: Increasing mortality with increasing weight.

The more fat that is eaten in the diet the greater is the risk of coronary heart disease. Fats are taken up from the intestines, enter the blood stream and are transported around the body. Fats are made up of several different substances. Those important in the development of heart disease are saturated fatty acids and cholesterol. Of the two, the level of cholesterol in the blood has been shown to be related to the risk of heart disease. Cholesterol is transported in the blood attached to fatty substances called lipoproteins. In many medical centres, middle-aged people are advised to have an annual blood test to measure their levels of plasma cholesterol, and those with raised levels are advised to alter their diet and to exercise more. Recently the measurements have become more sophisticated. It has been found that lipoprotein–cholesterol is not a single substance, but can be divided into fractions, depending on the density of the lipoprotein. The most important of these fractions are: high density lipoprotein–cholesterol (HDL–C); low density lipoprotein–cholesterol (LDL–C); and very low density lipoprotein–cholesterol (VDL–C). When the level of these subgroups was correlated with the risk of heart disease, it became apparent that a rise in LDL–cholesterol increased the risk of a heart attack, while a rise in HDL–cholesterol decreased the risk.

In other words, HDL–C is the good cholesterol and LDL–C is the bad cholesterol. The reason why LDL–C is the bad cholesterol is that it is involved in the narrowing of the arteries, particularly those supplying the muscles of the heart (the coronary arteries). The arteries become narrower because patches of lipid rich material (mostly LDL–C) are deposited under their inner lining. Over the years the patches increase in size and their surface becomes roughened. The roughened surface becomes covered by blood platelets, which leads to a clot forming. This blocks the artery further. If the blood flow is completely blocked a heart attack occurs.

HDL–C is the good cholesterol because it takes cholesterol out of the tissues and returns it to the liver where it is dealt with.

To determine the risk of a woman having a heart attack, many doctors recommend that women over the age of 40 should consider having their blood cholesterol measured. If the blood cholesterol is raised (greater than 6.2 mmol/L), the doctor may suggest to the woman that the subgroups of lipids in the blood, HDL–C and LDL–C, are measured so that the doctor can better advise the woman what she should do.

It is important that the tests should be interpreted carefully as the level of HDL–C falls and that of LDL–C rises with increasing age, and the change is most marked after a woman's menopause, because of the abrupt diminution in the secretion of oestrogen, rather than because she is growing older.

The blood level of LDL–C also increases if a woman becomes obese, and diminishes if the diet contains more complex carbohydrates and fibre and less saturated fats ('the prudent diet'). HDL–C increases if a 'prudent diet' is eaten, if weight is reduced, if exercise is taken regularly and the person ceases to smoke.

Because of the belief that the sex hormones might influence HDL–C and LDL–C, several investigations have been made among menopausal women.

The research has shown that oestrogen given alone to women who have had their ovaries removed (oöphorectomy) or to postmenopausal women, leads to a reduction in LDL–C, and a rise in HDL–C.

The effect of oestrogen treatment on the woman's blood lipids is complicated by the fact that it is now usual to give a progestogen for at least 12 days each month in addition to oestrogen when treating menopausal symptoms.

The question that has to be answered is: 'Do progestogens affect blood lipids, and is the lipid level influenced by the type of progestogen and the dose prescribed?'

The results from many studies are inconsistent and confusing, partly because in the investigations larger doses of progestogen were given than are prescribed today and partly because of flawed methodology.

In the past, the treatment of menopausal symptoms was to take an oestrogen for 21 days and to add a fairly large dose of a progestogen for the last 7 to 10 days of the treatment course. After a hormone-free interval of 7 days, another course of hormones was started. These hormonal regimens led to a fall in the level of HDL and a variable increase in LDL levels.

Recently, the accepted regimen for treatment of menopausal symptoms has been altered. Most doctors now prescribe an oestrogen to be taken everyday without a break, or a patch every 3 days, or an implant of oestrogen every 6 months. If the woman has not had a hysterectomy, the doctor prescribes a small dose of a progestogen to be taken for 12 days each month to protect the woman against developing endometrial cancer. Studies with various combinations of oestrogen and progestogen show that the effect on blood lipids of progestogen used today is smaller than when the larger doses of progestogen were taken and can probably be ignored. And as mentioned on p. 70, the new generation progestogens, which have no effect on blood lipids, will probably replace the progestogens currently prescribed in hormonal replacement treatment.

The beneficial alterations in the blood lipid levels of postmenopausal women due to oestrogen suggested to some doctors that if menopausal women were prescribed oestrogen they would be protected against heart attacks. What is the evidence that this idea is true?

Fifteen papers about the beneficial effect of oestrogen in protecting a postmenopausal woman against a heart attack have been published in the past 5 years. These papers show that oestrogen taken by women after the menopause reduces the risk of a heart attack by about half, particularly amongst women who have a raised blood cholesterol or high blood pressure and who smoke. However, it should be noted that the reported beneficial effect of oestrogen relates to a time when oestrogen was used alone and when progestogens were not added for some days during the month. It is possible that the protective effect of oestrogen may be reduced because the progestogens may counteract the beneficial effect of oestrogen on blood lipids, although as just mentioned, recent studies show that this does not occur with the lower dose of progestogen currently prescribed, particularly if one of the new generation progestogens mentioned is prescribed.

There is evidence that only half of the beneficial effect of oestrogen is due to its effect on blood lipids reducing the level of LDL–C in the blood and preventing its accumulation in the patches in the arteries. Oestrogen also improves the blood flow through the arteries, probably by dilating the vessels, and may have a direct beneficial effect on the arteries by reducing the size of the atheromatous patches.

As we mentioned earlier, it should also be noted that the risk of women aged 50 to 64 having a heart attack is not great. Information from Australia and the USA shows that in any one year about 6 women per 1000 women in the age group 50–59 will have a heart attack and only 1 of these women will die each year as a result. If hormones are taken the risk of having a heart attack falls to about 3 per 1000 women each year, and the chance of dying from a heart attack falls to about 1 in every 2000 women, in other words a 50 per cent reduction. Of course as a woman grows older, the chance of having a heart attack increases.

### Reducing the risk of coronary heart disease

What should a woman do in her middle years to reduce the risk of developing heart disease?

- She should eat a healthy diet as described in Chapter 4. This diet increases the amount of complex carbohydrate (for example, bread), vegetables and fruit and reduces the amount of sugar and fat in the diet.
- She should cease smoking if she is a smoker.
- She should take regular enjoyable exercise (a brisk 30 minute walk three times a week is sufficient);
- She should have her blood pressure checked each year;
- She should reduce her weight if she is obese;
- After the menopause she should consider taking oestrogen (hormone replacement treatment), unless there is a reason for not using this treatment (see page 80). A matter of concern which has been expressed is the fear that the oestrogen may increase the risk of stroke. A recent study shows that it does not, and may even reduce the risk.

A woman in her middle years, and when elderly, who has not chosen to take hormone replacement treatment in her early menopausal years, can start taking the hormones at any age to reduce the risk that she will have a heart attack, which increases dramatically after the age of 65. Older women are prescribed a very small dose of oestrogen at first and, over the weeks, the dose is increased to an amount which is protective against heart disease. The reason for starting with a very small dose is that some older women are sensitive to the side-effects of oestrogen and their body has to become accustomed to the hormone.

## STROKE

As people grow older, particularly when they are in late middle-age and elderly, stroke becomes increasingly common. A stroke may be caused in several ways. In three quarters of cases, it is due to a blood clot blocking an artery supplying the brain, which may have been narrowed by atherosclerosis. In the other cases, the stroke is caused by a brain haemorrhage.

Strokes occur more commonly in people who have a high blood pressure, who are overweight, who smoke, or who have diabetes. A woman may reduce her chance of having a stroke by following the advice given for reducing the risk of heart attack.

## THE URINARY TRACT SYSTEM

Women are more likely to develop urinary symptoms than men. About 20 per cent of women aged between 20 and 50 are likely to have an attack of painful and frequent urination in any year, indicating a probable attack of cystitis. After the age of 50 and particularly after the menopause, urinary problems become more frequent, because of the deficiency of oestrogen which occurs. The lack of oestrogen may affect the functioning of the bladder or the urethra, causing symptoms of frequency of urination, and sometimes pain when urine is passed. The symptoms are those of cystitis, but examination of the urine shows no infection. Oestrogen given as a vaginal cream of pessary or hormone replacement treatment often relieves the problem.

More disturbing to many postmenopausal women is the onset of involuntary urinary leakage. The leakage may occur following sneezing, coughing, laughing or excitement, or may follow an uncontrollable urge to pass urine. The proportion of women who have involuntary leakage of urine (urinary incontinence) in an inappropriate place more than twice a month, increases from less than 5 per cent in women under the age of 35 to over 15 per cent in women over the age of 60, according to a survey made in England.

Studies in Sweden of the population of a city showed similar results. By the age of 65, 14 per cent of the women complained of urinary incontinence and in half of them, leakage of urine occurred every day. By the age of 80, one woman in four had urinary incontinence, over half leaking urine every day.

In the Netherlands, a study of 700 postmenopausal women in a medium-sized town showed that 27 per cent had urinary incontinence.

It is clear that a large number of older women in many countries suffer from an embarrassing complaint and most put up with the discomfort and the smell rather than seeking help. Studies have shown that two-thirds of women who have quite severe incontinence, delay seeking help because of embarrassment or because they believe that it is normal to leak urine as a woman grows older.

Some women cope with their problem by wearing pads when they go out. Some women stop taking exercise because this increases the chance of wetting themselves, and some, after a particularly embarrassing episode of incontinence, change their life style completely remaining reclusively at home and rarely going out.

As treatment is available this is a pity.

There are several varieties of urinary incontinence. Some women who have infection of the bladder are incontinent. Other women have 'stress' incontinence, which is due to an anatomical failure of the muscles around the outlet of the bladder to close, particularly when the woman is 'stressed', for example when she laughs or jumps. Other incontinent women have so-called 'urgency' incontinence. This is due to an overactive bladder, which contracts when it contains only a small amount of urine. Other women have a mixture of stress incontinence and urgency incontinence. In fact, nearly two-thirds of the Dutch women who reported having urinary incontinence had the mixed type.

Because of the social embarrassment of being 'wet' and the fact that treatment is available, a woman should consider going to see her doctor or attending a hospital. After taking a history to exclude medical causes of incontinence, and arranging for an examination of a specimen of the urine to exclude infection of the urinary tract, the doctor may make some relatively simple tests to reach a diagnosis (Table 11.1). If the woman has passed the menopause and is not using hormone replacement treatment, and the urine leakage is not too disturbing, the doctor may suggest that the woman takes oestrogen, preferably vaginally, for a month and learns pelvic floor exercises. These measures relieve or cure up to 25 per cent of women with urinary incontinence. Alternatively, the woman may choose or the doctor may consider it preferable for her to attend a special clinic where tests are made to establish the exact diagnosis. The tests are needed because the symptoms of the two types of incontinence tend to be similar.

The tests are neither painful nor frightening but may be a bit embarrassing, although new methods are being developed to reduce the embarrassment. First a small tube the size of a sausage is introduced painlessly into the woman's vagina and an ultrasound picture is taken to see if there is any evidence of weakness in the bladder or abnormalities of the genital organs. The woman is then asked to go into a separate room and to empty her bladder in privacy into a commode, which electronically measures the amount of urine which she passes. She then comes back and a further ultrasound examination is made to check if she has any urine left in her bladder. The doctor may then decide that she needs to have a further test made.

### Table 11.1: Coping with urinary leakage

We recommend that a woman who has this complaint should see her doctor.

The doctor will:
1. Take a history and examine the woman to find out if the cause of the incontinence is due a medical condition. A urine sample is examined to exclude infection of the urinary tract.
2. Ask the woman to complete a pad test. She drinks 500 ml of water, and then walks about, climbing stairs, for example. The pad is examined (and weighed) one hour later to determine the amount of urinary leakage.
3. If the woman is postmenopausal and the leakage is not too inconveniencing, and she agrees, she uses a vaginal cream or tablet every day for the period of a month. This will relieve or cure the problem in up to one quarter of women.
4. Pelvic floor exercises may also be undertaken by the woman during this time.
5. If the leakage is severe, the hormone treatment or the pelvic floor exercises do not relieve the symptoms, she should consider attending a special clinic so that the exact diagnosis can be established by special tests

---

This involves putting a narrow tube into her bladder (through her urethra), and another into her rectum (back passage). The tubes have electronic gadgets attached to them which record the pressure in the bladder and in the rectum. The bladder is then filled slowly with water through the tube, and the changes in pressure are recorded. The woman is asked to say when she feels the need to pass urine. When her bladder is full she is asked to stand up and may be asked to cough several times, when some urine may leak. She is then asked to empty her bladder completely by urinating, and the recordings continue to be made.

The ultrasound findings and the records made electronically are inspected and the diagnosis confirmed. This is important as the treatment of stress incontinence and urge incontinence are quite different.

In general, stress incontinence is treated with surgery, although often the 'pelvic floor exercises' (described in Table 11.2) are tried for a few months first. Studies in the USA suggest that the exercises relieve incontinence in a number of women. An alternative is for the woman to buy a set of 5 vaginal cones, each weighing a bit more than its predecessor. The woman inserts the cone into her vagina, and

**Table 11.2:** Pelvic floor exercises

---

These exercises help a person strengthen the muscles which act as a sling to keep the bladder, the genital organs and the rectum in their correct position.

You should try to do the exercises at least once an hour when you are awake for the rest of your life.

At first you may find the exercises a bit tiring but persevere and you will find them easy to do. The pelvic floor exercises only take about two minutes of each hour and could relieve your urinary problems.

The exercises are easy to learn. No one can detect that you are doing them so they may be done when you are watching TV, washing the dishes, cleaning the house, or at work.

The exercises have three components:

1. When sitting down, contract the pelvic floor muscles, as if you were trying to lift your genital organs from the seat. Hold the contraction as you count 5 slowly (5 seconds). Then relax. Repeat the exercise 10 times.
2. Stand up and contract the pelvic floor muscles as if you were trying to stop the flow of urine in midstream, or if you were tightening your vagina. Hold the contraction for 5 seconds. Then relax. Repeat the exercise 10 times.
3. Finally do a fast version of the exercises, contracting and relaxing every second for 10 times.

You can check your progress if you wish and can make sure that you are contracting the right muscles by inserting your finger into your vagina and feeling the strength of the contraction.

If you do the exercises as described, after a week or two you will be pleased with the improvement of the grip.

---

keeps it in for increasing periods of time. When she is able to keep it in for 1 hour, she changes it for a heavier cone. As well, postmenopausal women should take oestrogen either as a vaginal cream or pessary (preferably, but the hormone can be taken by mouth), as it may relieve the symptoms without the woman having to resort to surgery or to complicated 'conditioning' treatment. Surgical treatment is either to inject a substance through the vagina on either side of the lowest part (or neck), of the bladder to strengthen the supporting muscles, or by an operation which lifts the bladder neck upwards.

Urge incontinence is not helped by surgery, and most women need drugs to reduce the sensitivity of the bladder to being filled, and to learn bladder retraining exercises which help to increase the capacity of the bladder before the message to the brain to pass urine occurs. As mentioned earlier, oestrogen treatment should be tried in postmenopausal women, as well.

What most incontinent women need is to be able to contact a helpful doctor who can explain about and arrange for the urodynamic tests which may be needed to determine the type of incontinence. The doctor should be able to reassure the woman that the staff at the Urodynamic clinic will be helpful and will suggest the most appropriate treatment to stop the incontinence and permit the woman to lead a full and enjoyable life.

## THE GENITAL SYSTEM

In the middle years, particularly after the menopause, three main problems affect a woman's genital system. These are:
1. the woman may develop postmenopausal bleeding;
2. she may have a prolapse;
3. she may develop a cancer of her uterus or her ovaries.

### Post menopausal bleeding

A woman who takes progestogens as part of hormone replacement treatment expects to have a bleed at the end of or just after finishing the progestogen: if the bleeding occurs *at other times*, it requires investigation. The investigation includes performing a hysteroscope examination (see page 27) or taking an endometrial biospy; that is, the removal of a small sample of the endometrium, using an endometrial biospy instrument (Fig 11.3). The procedure takes place in the doctor's rooms and does not require a general anaesthetic. Instead, either no anaesthetic is given or a local anaesthetic is injected into the cervix of the uterus. The sampler is introduced into the uterus through the cervix and is rotated inside the cavity of the uterus to obtain a sample of the endometrium. Most women find the procedure only a little uncomfortable, but one woman in 4 finds it painful or very painful.

The specimen of the endometrium is sent for pathological examination and, provided no cancer is found, treatment is not usually needed.

Sometimes the doctor arranges for an ultrasound examination, as this give evidence that endometrial cancer is present, or arranges for the woman to have a hysteroscopy.

## Cancer

Most cancers become more common as a person grows older and cancers of the genital tract are no exception. Luckily, both cervical cancer and endometrial cancer can be detected early in a woman if she is prepared to be examined vaginally at regular intervals. As well, any woman who develops abnormal bleeding from her vagina (especially if she has passed her menopause), should go to a doctor so that genital tract cancer can be excluded.

This is where the Pap smear is so helpful. Warning cells, which may develop into cervical cancer, can be detected if a woman has a Pap smear every 2 years and a vaginal examination is made at the same time. Unfortunately many women in their middle years do not have regular Pap smears and when they do consult a doctor (usually because of vaginal bleeding), they may have developed a cervical cancer.

Endometrial cancer, as mentioned previously, usually shows itself by abnormal bleeding in the years after the menopause. As it grows slowly, in most cases a cure is likely. The important thing is for a postmenopausal woman not to delay seeing her doctor if she develops unexpected vaginal bleeding.

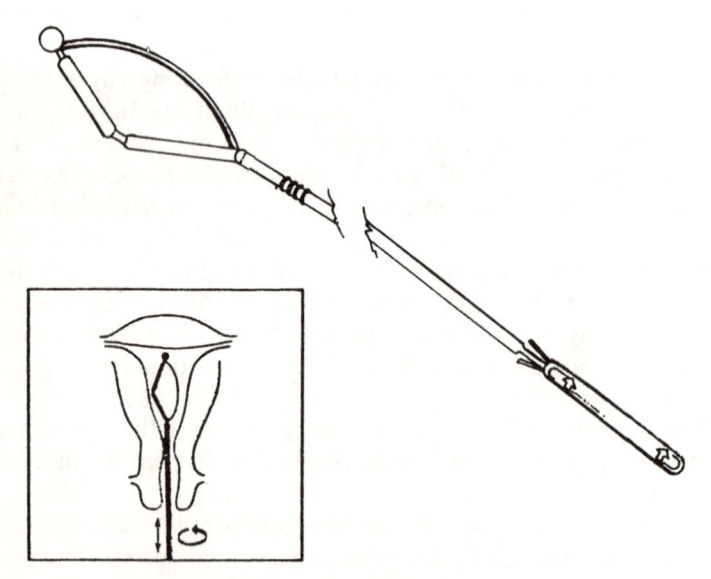

Figure 11.3:  Endometrial biopsy instrument.

Cancer of the ovary is a problem, because in most cases it cannot be detected until late in the disease. Some doctors recommend annual vaginal examinations and special blood tests to try to detect the cancer, but studies show that neither of these measures is very helpful. Research is continuing to try to find a way of detecting ovarian cancer at a curable stage.

## Prolapse

A woman entering the postmenopausal years, who has given birth one or more times, has an increased chance of developing a prolapse. A prolapse is due to the tissues, particularly the muscles of the pelvis which support and keep the vagina and the uterus in their normal positions in the body, stretching so that the vagina or the uterus or both fall downwards. If the front wall of the vagina is poorly supported by the muscles of the pelvis, the wall and the bladder which lie close to it may bulge into the entrance to the vagina, particularly when the woman strains to pass urine. If the posterior wall of the vagina is not well supported by the muscles of the pelvis, it may prolapse, carrying down the rectum, so that it bulges and can be seen at the vulva. These types of prolapse may occur independently, or the uterus may prolapse down the vagina as well. This is due to a lack of support by the ligaments and muscles which normally hold the uterus in its position (Fig. 11.4).

Following childbirth, many women have mild degrees of prolapse, but after the menopause the prolapse may become more obvious and may cause discomfort as the woman feels pressure in her vagina and that 'something is coming down'.

The cause of prolapse is that during childbirth, the supporting tissues are stretched and are not so strong as before the birth. Over the years they become weaker and prolapse occurs. With better care during childbirth, the number of women complaining of prolapse has diminished, but the problem has not gone away. The reason why prolapse becomes more frequent after the menopause is because the lack of oestrogen reduces the blood supply to the supporting tissues, so that their strength is further reduced.

From this description, it is evident that the prevention of uterovaginal prolapse should start after childbirth, when the exercises (shown in Table 11.2) to strengthen the supporting tissues should be started. Many women have not been told about these exercises after giving birth; other women find them boring to do and forget to do them.

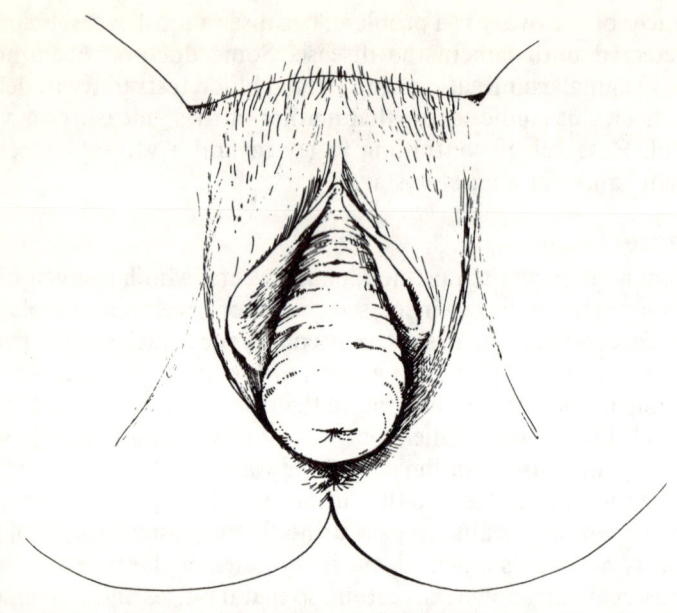

Figure 11.4: Uterine prolapse. The supports holding the uterus in position have weakened and the cervix now protrudes through the vagina when the woman stands or strains.

Although the pelvic floor exercises may help when a prolapse is noticed in a woman's middle years, many women who have a prolapse will decide to have surgery. The type of surgery depends on the doctor's assessment of the degree of prolapse and the woman's wishes. For example, a prolapse which involves both the vagina and the uterus may be treated by removing the uterus vaginally (vaginal hysterectomy), and repairing the stretched tissues of the vagina, or by strengthening the supports of the uterus (thus avoiding a hysterectomy).

Some women may be concerned that the surgery may make enjoyable sexual intercourse painful. This should not happen if the gynaecologist who operates is skilled in vaginal surgery.

## THE BREASTS

In the reproductive years, between 15 and 49, the glandular tissues in a woman's breasts are stimulated each month by the hormones secreted by her ovaries. Most women know that in the week or ten days before menstruation their breasts become fuller, sometimes tender and occasionally painful. A few women have painful breasts which persist through the month. Although several treatments have been tried for the condition, which is called benign breast disease, in about 20 per cent of affected women none of the treatments works.

As the menopause approaches, the breasts symptoms tend to become less, to the delight of women who have benign breast disease, but in a few women the symptoms may persist or even get more severe. Once the menopause has occurred, the hormones secreted by the ovaries cease to be produced, and the glandular tissue of the breasts decreases in size. The breasts often get smaller, but as the glandular tissue only makes up a small portion of the breasts of women who have large breasts (fatty tissue makes up most of the rest), the breasts may remain the same size or even increase in size.

Although the glandular tissue of the breast becomes relatively inactive after the menopause, breast cancer may develop in it. Breast cancer is the most common site of cancer in women. One woman in every 15 will develop breast cancer some time in her life, usually after the age of 50.

Breast cancer can only be cured if it is detected at an early stage. For this reason some form of breast examination at regular intervals has been recommended for all women, especially those nearing the menopause, and those in their postmenopausal years.

There are three ways of examining the breasts — breast self examination, breast examination by a doctor and mammography.

## Breast self examination (BSE)

In the past 30 years the notion has arisen that if a woman examined her breasts each month from about the age of 25, any lump that had developed would be detected early. If the lump turned out to be a breast cancer, the early detection would lead to a better chance of cure.

Most national cancer societies have promoted breast self examination (BSE) as have many doctors and some women's groups. For example the Boston Women's Health Collective in their book: *The New Our Bodies: Ourselves*, wrote that they believe that women are the best monitors of their own breasts and probably will be able to detect an abnormality better than many doctors who have to take into account the wide variation in the breasts of different women, which they examine only once or twice a year. Women are also concerned that 'most doctors are trained to discredit what patients, particularly women, report about themselves'.

Studies by doctors about the value of BSE have been few and have been retrospective, that is they have asked women who have developed breast cancer whether they practised BSE or not, or have checked whether BSE increased the survival rate of women who had breast cancer. The results of these studies show that BSE is less effective in the early detection of breast cancer than examination by a trained doctor or by mammography.

There was also concern that BSE might cause considerable anxiety to women who detected a lump or some other abnormality in one of their breasts. This opinion was well expressed by two Canadian physicians in 1985, who concluded that BSE might do more harm than good, especially in women under the age of 40. The breasts of women under the age of 40 respond more readily to the fluctuating hormone levels that occur during the menstrual cycle, and may develop transient lumps. If a lump was discovered and the doctor consulted was not skilled in breast examination, an unnecessary operation might be recommended.

Whilst this could happen, most health professionals agree that breast self examination (or breast self awareness, as some people call it) has benefits which exceed the problems which it might occasion. Most recommend that a woman (or her partner if she prefers) should examine her breasts several times a year in the week after her menstrual period and, after the age of 30 should consider visiting a doctor once a year for a breast examination. This is considered later in this chapter.

The reason for terming the examination, breast self awareness, recognizes that women are often reluctant to examine their breasts, and aims to change this.

Breast self examination is not difficult. A woman can do it easily if she follows these steps (provided by the Anti Cancer Council of Victoria).

*Step 1:* Stand in front of a mirror, put your hands by your side and look at your breasts. Then raise your hands above your head and look again. Now put your hands on your hips, press firmly, elbows forward (which puts the chest [pectoral] muscles on a stretch), and look again. You are looking at your breasts to see if the shape of each has changed since your last self examination; if any part of the skin is puckered; if there is a bulge or a flattened area in the breast; or if either nipple has been drawn into the breast tissue.

# THE MIDDLE YEARS AND THE BODY SYSTEMS

*Step 2: Getting into position:* If your breasts are small, you can examine them lying down or in the shower.

If they are medium to large, you should examine them lying down. This position spreads your breast as thinly as possible, which makes you more likely to detect a lump, even a very small one.

Let's begin with your *right* breast.

*The lying-down position:* First, lie on your left side with your knees bent. Now, roll back so that your shoulders are flat on the bed — but don't move your legs. Put your right arm under your head.

If your breasts are very large, place a pillow under your right shoulder.

Your breast is now spread as flat as possible.

*The standing position:* If you are small-breasted, you can do BSE in the shower, using soap to help your fingers slide easily over your skin.

To examine your right breast stand with your right arm behind your head (Fig. 11.5a).

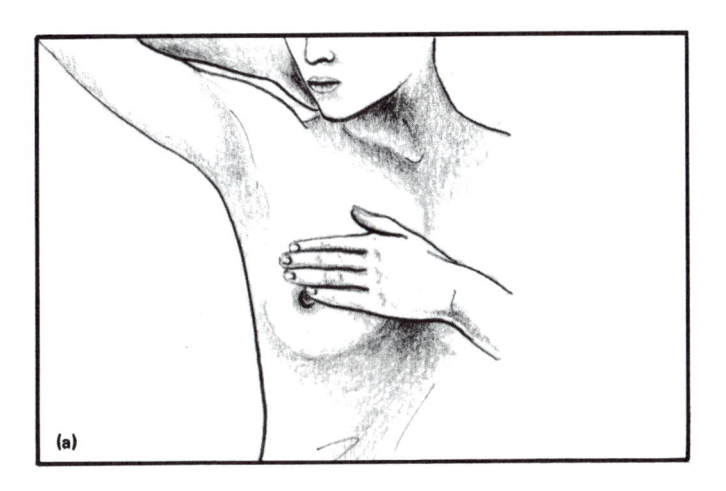

Figure 11.5a

*Step 3: Starting your BSE:* You examine all the breast area following an imaginary line of vertical 'strips' starting in your armpit and working up and down across your breast.

You use the flat part of your fingers including the sensitive finger pads. You work in small circles about 5 centimetres across. Use the diagram shown in Figure 11.5b to practise.

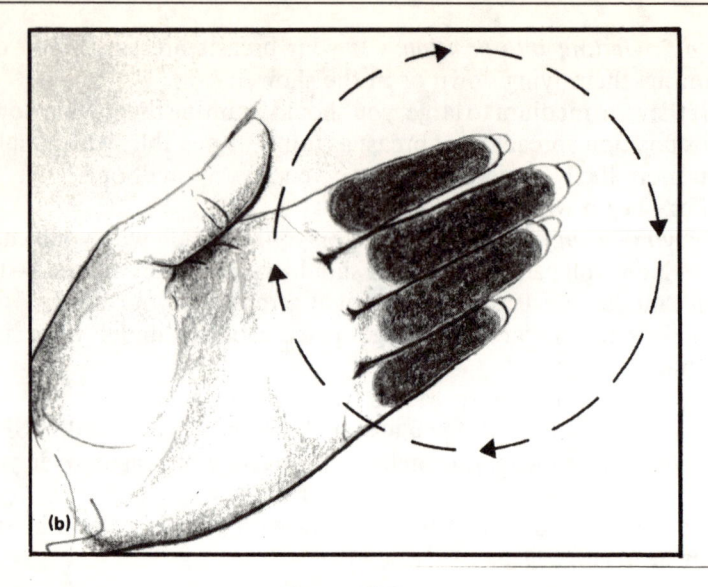

Figure 11.5b

At *each* spot you touch, you should use *two pressures* — *lightly* and then *firmly*.
*Feel lightly:* With your fingers together and flat, make the first circle with a light pressure, firm enough to make a slight 'dent' in your skin (Fig. 11.5c).

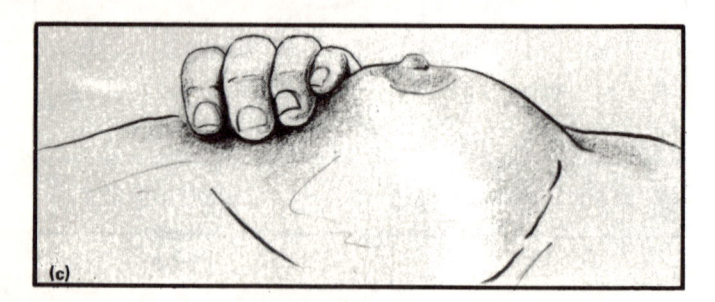

Figure 11.5c

You are feeling for anything near the surface of your skin.
*Feel firmly:* At the *same* spot, make a second circle pressing quite firmly, so you can feel any lump *deep* in your breast. Press as firmly as you can without discomfort (Fig. 11.5d). Most women can feel their ribs with this firm pressure.

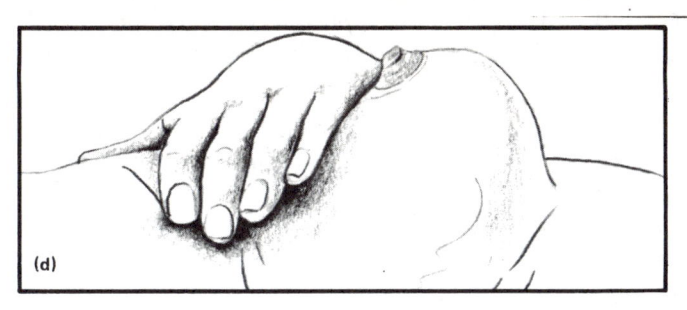

Figure 11.5d

Now proceed as follows: Using your *left* hand, begin the first 'strip' at your armpit. Make a circle of light, and then of firm pressure at this first spot. Move your hand gradually towards the bra-line, using circles of light and firm pressure at *each* spot.

At the bottom of the bra-line, move across about 2 centimetres to the left and start working upwards to your collar bone, making circles all the time.

Work up and down your breast in strips until you reach your nipple (Fig. 11.5e).

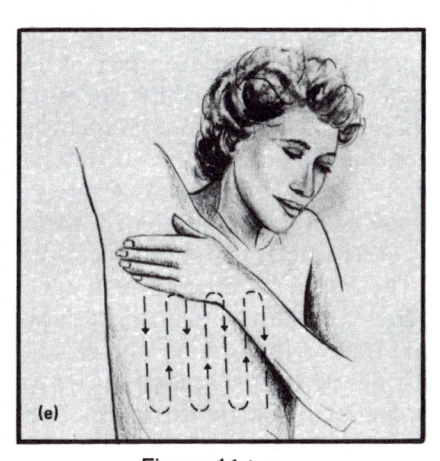

Figure 11.5e

*Step 4: Changing position:* When you reach the nipple, lie flat on your back. This flattens the inner half of your breast. (If doing BSE in the shower, you don't need to change position).

Complete the nipple strip and continue the circles moving up and down in strips.

Remember the *light and firm pressures* at *each* spot.

Examine all the breast until you have completed the last strip between your breasts.

*Step 5: Checking your armpit:* Bring your right arm down by your side and feel your armpit firmly. Again you're looking for any lumps.

Now start again, at Step 2, and repeat the procedure for your *left* breast.

*Lying down position:* Lie on your *right* side, roll back so your shoulders are flat. Put your *left* arm behind your head.

*Standing position:* Stand with your left arm behind your head. Use your *right* hand to examine your *left* breast.

## Regular examinations by a health professional

Many authorities, including the national cancer societies in several countries, recommend that a woman should have a breast examination performed by a trained health professional, at regular intervals. The American Cancer Society, for example, recommended in 1980 that women aged 20 to 40 should have breast examinations at 3-yearly intervals, and from the age of 40 onwards the breast examination should be performed annually. The technique of breast examination used by the trained examiner is identical to that used for breast self examination but the examiner additionally examines the armpit for evidence of enlarged lymph nodes. The recognition of the importance of regular breast examination by health professionals has led to the establishment of 'Breast Clinics' in hospitals or as free-standing clinics in city areas. Many women, mostly from the affluent section of society, are prepared to visit these institutions, but many other women are afraid of going to a hospital or to a special clinic. Their need for breast screening is as great.

Most women do not need to go to a special breast clinic as many family doctors are trained to examine women's breasts, and many women visit their family doctor at least once a year. The woman needs only to ask the family doctor to examine her breasts, or if she prefers, go to a community health clinic and be examined there by a health professional.

It must be said that the effectiveness of breast examination in the detection of breast lumps and their interpretation depends on the skill of the examiner. A recent study shows that some doctors miss or misinterpret breast lumps. This finding and the relative

Table 11.3: Guidelines for detecting breast cancer

* If a woman detects a lump in her breast she should see a doctor urgently so that its nature can be determined.
* A woman who has no breast problems and who is aged 25 or older should examine her breasts every month following a menstrual period or if she has reached the menopause every month about the same time.
* A woman who has no breast problems and who is aged 35 should have her breasts examined by a doctor every 3 years; and women over the age of 40 should have an annual breast examination.
* A woman who has no breast symptoms and who is aged 35 to 40 years should have a 'base line' mammogram, with which subsequent mammograms can be compared.
* A woman who has no breast symptoms and who is aged between 40 and 50 should consult with her doctor about the need for an annual mammogram. For example, women who have a mother or a sister who has had breast cancer, or who are childless or whose first child was born after the age of 35, probably should have annual mammograms from the age of 40.
* A woman who has no breast problems and who is aged 50 and over should have a mammogram each year.

crudeness of breast examination has led some doctors to suggest that an annual breast examination might be replaced by screening by mammography of all women over the age of 40.

Other doctors do not think that this is a good idea, as 40 per cent of breast cancers are first detected by the woman herself (who feels a lump in her breasts), or by her doctor. The best approach is for women to perform breast self examination each month, to have an annual breast check by a doctor and if she is over the age of 45 (earlier if a close relative has had breast cancer), to have regular mammograms (Table 11.3).

Mammography

A mammogram is a special X-ray picture of the breasts, which uses a very low dose of radiation to obtain the picture (Fig. 11.6). Careful investigations have shown that mammography is safe for women over the age of 40 and does not induce cancer even when an annual mammogram is made.

In 1971, a randomized trial of mammography was reported from New York. This trial showed that deaths from breast cancer were reduced among those screened, although some unnecessary

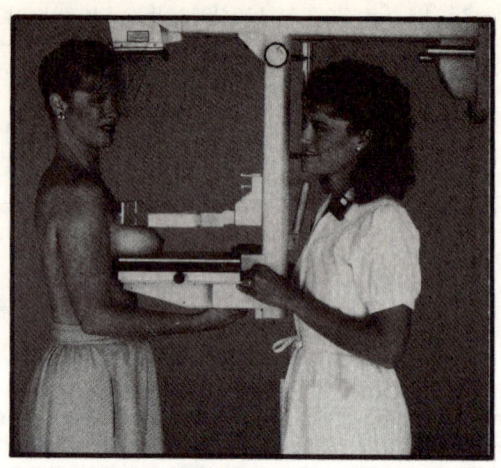

**Figure 11.6** A patient and radiographer using a mammography unit (Reproduced by kind permission of Laserex Medicon and Xerox U.K.)

operations, including mastectomy, were performed. Later, more carefully organized studies have been reported from Sweden and the Netherlands. These studies show that mammography, using today's techniques, detects breast cancer at an earlier stage than the older methods of mammography.

The studies show that nearly 60 per cent of breast cancers can be detected by mammography at a stage when breast examination by a doctor fails to find them, as the cancer is so small. Other research shows that if 70 per cent of women aged 50 and over had regular mammograms, there would be a 25 to 35 per cent reduction in deaths from this common cancer.

The value of mammography in women over the age of 40 is that it is easy to perform, and that it may detect a breast cancer before it can be detected clinically. The disadvantages of mammography are that a suspicious finding does not necessarily indicate that there is breast cancer. In about ten women in every 1000 examined, the mammogram will detect a suspicious area. It is important to know that only two suspicious areas in every ten detected by mammography, turn out to be breast cancer after biopsy.

Current recommendations are that a 'base line' mammogram should be made when the woman is aged about 40 and thereafter every 2 years to the age of 50 and then annually.

There are certain problems about adopting this advice. At present, fewer than 25 per cent of women aged 50 ever have a mammogram, and fewer than 5 per cent have an annual mammogram. If every woman aged 50 or more had a mammogram each year, the cost would be great and there are insufficient radiographers to make the picture and insufficient radiologists to interpret it. As well, a suspicious mammogram means that further investigations are needed. These usually consist of an examination of the breast by an experienced doctor and, often, an ultrasound picture to determine more precisely the nature of the suspicious area detected. A narrow needle may be introduced into the suspicious area by the specialist and a sample of tissue removed for laboratory diagnosis. One woman in 15 needs to attend for a second mammogram or for further investigation. One woman in 50 needs to have a minor operation to remove the suspicious area. The woman usually only needs to remain in the hospital for a few hours. The doctor makes a small curved incision along one of the 'tension lines of the breast'. He then dissects carefully until the area is reached. He then excises it. Healing is quick and the scar is almost invisible after a few months.

As these procedures take time and are costly, the problems mount. Clearly experts and consumers need to discuss the problems and suggest remedies.

It is important that the woman has the opportunity to talk about her fears if a suspicious area is detected by the mammogram, as usually a few days elapse before further investigations are made. Most mammography screening programmes provide this service. Some women are worried that the amount of radiation required for annual mammograms may increase the risk of developing a cancer somewhere in the body. These woman can be reassured. Recent studies show that the increased risk from mammographic screening is less than one in a million.

## THYROID DISEASE

About 1.5 per cent of women of all ages have deficiency of thyroid hormone (hypothyroidism), and after the age of 60, the proportion rises to about 5 per cent.

Testing for thyroid deficiency is the third most common laboratory test made in many Western countries. This is because doctors believe that women (and men) who complain of fatigue, lethargy, slow thinking, feeling cold, a dry skin, and whose mood is 'flat' may have hypothyroidism. The tests are simple. A sample of blood is drawn and two hormones, thyroid stimulating hormone and thyroxine are measured.

If the woman is found to be hypothyroid she is given tablets of thyroxine. Thyroxine may not be a harmless preparation, and the dose should be monitored carefully, because high blood levels of thyroxine may increase the risk that the woman will develop osteoporosis, particularly if the hormone has been taken for a long time. For example, two groups of scientists independently found that amongst premenopausal women who had been taking thyroxine for five years or more, the density of the neck of their thigh bone (femur), was 13 per cent lower than that of women of their age who were not taking thyroxine. In other words they were at risk of developing osteoporosis.

Their recommendation was that women who have been diagnosed as having hypothyroidism should have their thyroid hormones tested at regular intervals, and that the dose of thyroxine should be adjusted to maintain the levels in the normal range.

# 12

# A WOMAN'S SKIN IN HER MIDDLE YEARS

*There is no magician's mantle to compare with the skin in its diverse roles of waterproof, overcoat, sunshade, suit of armour and refrigerator, sensitive to the touch of a feather, to temperature and pain, withstanding the wear and tear of three score years and ten, and executing its own running repairs.*

So wrote the anatomist R. D. Lockhart in a description that could hardly be bettered.

The skin varies in thickness, being only 0.5 mm thick on the eyelids and 4 mm thick, or more, on the soles of the feet. In places, such as the palms of the hands and the ears, it is firmly bound to the underlying structures. In other places, it is freely moveable. It is smooth or rough, dry or moist, depending on the number of sweat and sebaceous glands it contains. Most of it is covered with hairs, which may be soft and downy, scarcely perceptible, or may be coarse and long. In youth, the skin is firm and elastic; in age it is often loose and wrinkled. It holds a mirror to health and to age, changing in its appearance.

This vital organ, 1.7 square metres in extent, covers the body, protecting and isolating it from the environment. The skin consists of two layers, the outer layer, the epidermis, and the inner layer, the dermis, and both are of equal importance. The epidermis, which interfaces with the environment, is made up of layers of cells all of which are derived from the deepest layer. As the cells mature, they change in shape and in character, until near the surface they lose their nuclei and become a horny layer. From this layer, which varies in thickness, dead cells are constantly shed — over 9 g being lost each day, mostly invisibly, but sometimes embarrassingly as

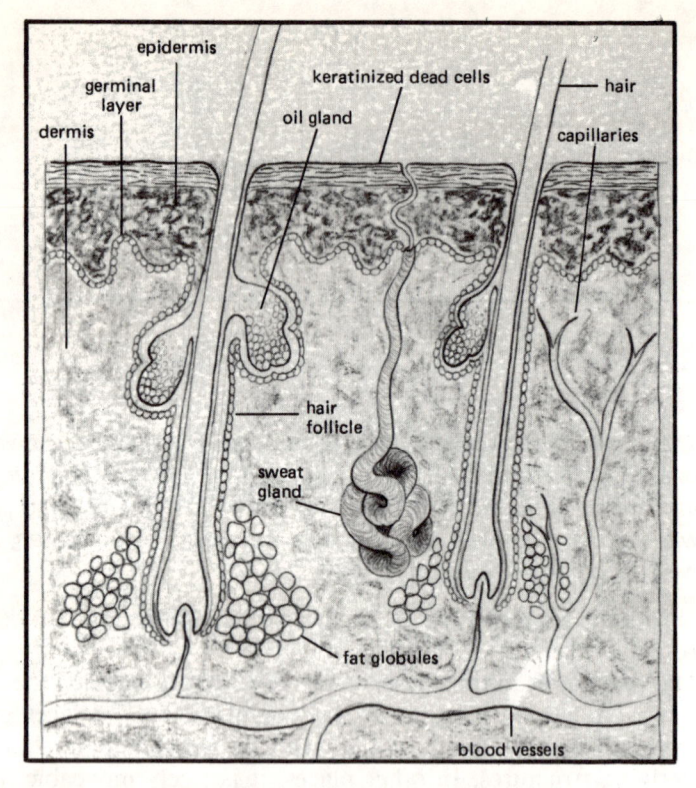

Figure 12.1: The structure of the skin

dandruff. This horny layer is vital for life because it is the waterproof layer of the skin. However, certain medications, hormones and poisons can enter the body through the skin, so its waterproofing is not perfect.

The pigmentation of the skin is due to tiny particles of a substance called melanin in the deepest layers of the epidermis. The more melanin, the darker the skin. Melanin protects the skin against the damaging effects of sunlight, which is why 'white'-skinned people tan when exposed to sunlight, but, unfortunately, the skin itself may be damaged, although the tissues beneath it are protected.

The dermis is a felted meshwork of fibrous and elastic tissues, which is riveted to the epidermis by projections that stud its surface (Fig. 12.1). The fibrous tissue is mainly formed from a protein called collagen. In the dermis are found the roots of the hairs, with their accompanying sebaceous glands and the sweat glands, all of which open on the skin's surface through narrow tubes.

The skin is a restless organ, constantly rearranging itself, constantly shedding surface cells and making new cells. Through it hairs grow, which increase in length, live for about 2 years and are then replaced by new hairs growing from the hair follicle deep in the dermis. The sebaceous glands are constantly active, secreting the oil-like sebum, which is similar to the lanolin of sheep's wool, and which greases the surface of the body, keeping the skin pliable. If the gland making sebum becomes blocked, a whitehead, a blackhead or a small cyst will result.

With the passage of the years, and the assaults of the environment, the appearance of the skin changes. The epidermis becomes thinner, drier and may become flaky, particularly in cold climates in winter. The legs are often affected and the flakiness is aggravated by overheated houses in which the relative humidity is low. The reason for the increased rate of shedding of the outer cells of the skin is not understood, but may be related to a reduction in the thickness of the skin with age, and in very old people the skin may become parchment-like and almost transparent.

As a person grows older, the melanin granules, which respond to sunlight by multiplying, become fewer and respond less efficiently, so that skin cancer is likely to become more common.

The dermis also changes as a person ages. It provides support for the tissues lying above and below it and is responsible for the resilience and elasticity of the skin. As a person grows older, a change occurs in the superficial part of the dermis — the elastic fibres become shorter and the meshwork becomes discontinuous.

As well, an alteration occurs in the amount and the integrity of the second type of fibre in the skin, the collagen fibres. The effect of these changes, which begin at about the age of 30, is that fine wrinkles and lines appear on the skin exposed to the sunlight, and the skin under the chin and on the upper arms and legs may become lax and stretched.

The collagen fibres seem to be the most important supporting fibres. The quantity of collagen in the skin is thought to be related to the 'quality' of the skin. The less collagen there is, the fewer elastic fibres are present and the more likely are wrinkles to be found. It has been shown that, from the age of 30, the amount of collagen in the skin decreases by about 1 per cent each year. It decreases rather more rapidly in women than in men, and it is believed that testosterone, the male hormone, protects a man's skin.

Another change in ageing skin is that the elastic fibres tend to become fewer after the menopause. This also suggests that oestrogen helps to protect the skin from the ravages of time and of the sun.

Ageing in the exposed skin is influenced considerably by climatic factors, particularly exposure to the sun's ultraviolet light. Ultra-violet light, over a period of time, damages the tissues, causing a break-up of collagen and elastic fibres. The degree to which the sun damages the skin depends on the person's heredity. It occurs less frequently in black races, whose skin is protected by the greater amount of melanin in it, and in certain families of white races.

The changes in the non-exposed parts of the skin are due, mainly, to the alteration in content and distribution of collagen, a reduction in elastic fibres, and a loss of water from the cells that make up the skin. This makes the skin loose and 'saggy'.

The changes in skin have been described at some length as many women attribute the changes in the skin to the menopause. It is certain that this is not so.

Most women in our society would prefer to remain slim, beautiful, with good skin, few wrinkles and glistening hair, well into middle-age.

In this situation, it was to be expected that someone would suggest that hormones might be involved; after all, menopausal women tend to have some wrinkles and as the woman moves into the menopausal years, the wrinkles tend to increase. As oestrogen levels in the blood fall after the menopause, when wrinkles increase, is it not likely that the two findings are connected?

## OESTROGEN AND THE SKIN

Does oestrogen improve the quality of the skin and prevent wrinkles?

The evidence that oestrogen increases the thickness of the skin, and makes it more youthful, is confused. A group of doctors in Finland and another in Britain have claimed that oestrogen has this effect. However, a comparable study carried out by another group of doctors in England failed to find that oestrogen, either as tablets or as a skin cream, prevented wrinkles. However, oestrogen may make them less obvious in three ways. First, oestrogen reduces the rate of collagen loss from the skin. Second, oestrogen increases the water content of the skin. Third, it may improve blood flow through the blood vessels in the dermis, which would have the effect of increasing the fluid retained in the skin. The three changes induced by oestrogen would prevent the skin from becoming thin and would tend to make wrinkles less obvious. But, alas, oestrogen does not make a dry skin less dry.

If oestrogen treatment does not make much difference to a menopausal woman's skin, is there anything that she can do? Clearly she cannot reverse the changes that have occurred, but she can improve the dry skin that becomes common as a woman grows older.

Cosmetic manufacturers have noted the concern of many women about their skins and offer a bewildering range of 'skin foods', lotions and creams that 'moisturize' dry skin and keep it youthful.

'Skin foods' perhaps have the largest impact. Large numbers of women, persuaded by skilled advertising, purchase creams, lotions, skin tonics and hormone preparations to delay the ageing process in the skin. The products are lavishly launched, superbly packaged, seductively perfumed, and are often very expensive. Do they do what they purport to do; namely, delay the inevitable changes that occur in the skin as a woman ages? The answer is that they do not. The best way to keep the skin in good condition is by cleaning it regularly using soap and water and drying it carefully. There is no cosmetic that will keep a woman's skin youthful if her genetic inheritance decrees that it ages quickly. The skin may be abused in youth by excessive sunbathing, which will hurry the ageing process (and may also cause skin cancer), but it is unlikely that the moisturizing creams that are purchased to limit the effects of that abuse are of any more benefit than the use of a cheap vaseline or lanolin product. Vaseline or lanolin will help the skin to look smooth and soft, and are just as effective as a more expensive moisturizer.

Moisturizers help dry skin, but the effectiveness of the moisturizer bears no relationship to its cost, according to a survey made by the Australian Consumers' Association, (ACA) after studying 72 cosmetic products. The survey showed that there was no relationship between the effectiveness of the product, the user's age, the climatic conditions or the user's skin type. According to the ACA this means that you waste money if you buy a moisturizer that is especially expensive, or said to be for 'mature skin', or for special weathers or seasons, or especially for 'combination' skin, unless you want to

**Table 12.1:** Moisturizers

*For a light lotion:*
    100 g sorbolene (with 10 per cent glycerine)
    500 ml of hot water
    (0.6 g benzoic acid if required)
    1.5–2.0 ml of perfume essence (if required)

*For a heavy lotion/light cream:*
    100 g sorbolene (with 10 per cent glycerine)
    300 ml of hot water
    (0.4 g benzoic acid if required)
    1.5–2.0 ml perfume essence (if required)

*For a mousse-type cream:*
    100 g sorbolene (with 10 per cent glycerine)
    150 ml of hot water
    (0.25 g benzoic acid if required)
    1.5–2.0 ml perfume essence (if required)

*For a heavier cream:*
    100 g sorbolene (with 10 per cent glycerine)
    100 ml of hot water
    (0.2 g benzoic acid if required)
    1.5–2.0 ml perfume essence (if required)

Courtesy of the Australian Consumers' Association

indulge yourself or give yourself a 'lift'. Nor are night creams any more effective than other moisturizers.

The survey confirmed that an effective moisturizer used night and morning after thorough cleansing of the face improves the condition of the skin for about 6 weeks and then maintains its condition.

A commercial skin moisturizer can be bought but it is much cheaper to make one at home. The Australian Consumers' Association (ACA) offers do-it-yourself moisturizers, which prove as effective as any of the commercial products (Table 12.1). ACA found that sorbolene with glycerine (and perfume if desired) is as effective as any of the commercial preparations and is considerably cheaper. Sorbolene (cetomacrogol cream) is a basic non-prescription skin cream, which many dermatologists recommend to patients who are allergic to perfume. Basically it consists of 10 per cent propylene glycerol (a moistener), 15 per cent of a non-ionic emulsifier (and 0.1 per cent preservative if required), made up in water.

Sorbolene with 10 per cent added glycerine makes a pleasant hand lotion, and it is recommended by ACA as a moisturizer, when made up in the following way. 'The basic method is simple. The sorbolene containing 10 per cent added glycerine (and benzoic acid dissolved in alcohol, only if required as a preservative) is placed in a bowl, and about 100 ml of the hot water added (distilled water may be used if preferred). The mixture is beaten with an old-fashioned egg-beater (we found this better than a processor). The rest of the hot water is added and the mixture beaten again. Perfume essence, if required, can be beaten into the mixture after it has cooled.' The quantities to be used are given in Table 12.1. The moisturizer should be stored in screw-top containers in the fridge, and small quantities removed as needed. An alternative way of preserving the cream is to add benzoic acid dissolved in alcohol (which will need to be made up by a pharmacist). If boiled or distilled water is used to make the lotion, the chance of contamination by bacteria is reduced.

## PHOTOAGED SKIN

The changes in the skin which occur with increasing age are different from the changes which inevitably occur with age. Skin is damaged by shorter ultraviolet light over the years. This light damages the connective tissue and the collagen in the dermis so that the skin has areas of thickness, irregularity and pigmented patches (as the small vessels in the skin may also be damaged).

It has been found that a drug called tretinoin (Airol, Retin–A), which is used to treat severe acne, may also restore skin damaged by excessive exposure to the sun ('photoaged'). A pea-sized quantity of tretinoin is applied to the face and neck every evening. In the first week of treatment the cream is left on the skin for 2 hours, in the next week the time is increased to 4 hours, and thereafter applied at night and washed off the next morning. During the first weeks of treatment nearly all the women complain of stinging, redness and peeling of the skin, but these symptoms settle in 1 to 3 months.

After 3 months treatment, a noticeable improvement of the skin occurs with less mottling and wrinkling, and better tone and tightness. However, the treatment has to be continued for at least a year or more to obtain the best effects, and probably should be continued for life. Each morning the woman should apply a little moisturizer to the face and neck. If the person goes out in the sun, she should use a 15+ sunscreen, as tretinoin may sensitize the skin to sunlight.

Further studies are needed before this treatment can be recommended but it may be a positive step to improving photodamaged skin.

## OESTROGEN AND THE HAIR

Does oestrogen improve the quality of the hair?

Growth of hair on the body, in both men and women, depends on the blood levels of a special form of the male hormone, testosterone. A few men lack the enzyme that converts testosterone into this special form and they have hairless bodies. Oestrogen tends to reduce hair growth, but does not influence its quality or quantity. There is no evidence that if oestrogen is given to menopausal women, they will have glistening, healthy hair.

# 13

# THE MIND IN A WOMAN'S MIDDLE YEARS

There is a belief by many women and many doctors that the menopause is associated with a deterioration in a woman's mental capacity, her ability to reason and to make deductions, and her feeling of 'well being'. The belief is not new. It was reported in the nineteenth-century and in 1901 an American Professor of Obstetrics and Gynaecology, Dr Florence Dressler, wrote in her book *Feminology — A Guide for Womankind* that during the menopause

> 'the once happy woman becomes despondent, moody and taciturn. She avoids company, has no taste for amusements and spends her time in watching the various symptoms, and bewailing her real and imaginary woes. In many cases, actual insanity, usually of a temporary nature, is the result of the disturbances which her system undergoes at this time'.

Twenty five years later, a British physician, Leonard Williams, in a book entitled *Middle Age and Old Age* wrote,

> 'But whatever the physical diseases or ailments the climacteric may be said to dispose the patient, it is upon her brain that the weight of the disorder usually falls ... It is common for the subjective sensations to be so overwhelming as to produce, or at any rate be accompanied by, such a degree of general irritability and unreasonableness as to render the patient increasingly difficult and eventually impossible'.

The belief that many women became mentally distressed during the menopause was confirmed by psychiatrists and given the approval of the American Psychiatric Association which, in 1968, declared that many menopausal women suffered from what they called 'involutional melancholia'. This was defined as 'a disorder occurring in the involutional period and characterized by worry, anxiety, agitation, and severe insomnia. Feelings of guilt and somatic preoccupations are frequently present and may be of delusional proportions. This disorder is distinguishable from manic depressive illness by the absence of previous episodes ... and it is distinguishable from psychotic depressive reaction in that the depression is not due to some life experience'.

Although the term 'involutional melancholia' was abandoned by the American Psychiatric Association in 1978, for a century and a half doctors believed that many menopausal women complained of 'mental' symptoms such as depression, irritability, anxiety, nervousness, fatigue, poor concentration, and headaches.

While it is true that some menopausal women complain of some of these symptoms, they are experienced at all ages and by both sexes, although women are more likely to seek help for 'anxiety or depression' than are men, perhaps because there are fewer ways in which women can obtain relief from unhappiness, or stress than men.

As the psychological symptoms are experienced by both sexes and at all ages, they cannot be part of a 'menopausal syndrome'. This is borne out by several studies. For example, one measure of the degree of psychiatric problems occurring in the years around the menopause is the frequency of first admissions to psychiatric hospitals. In Figure 13.1 it can be seen that fewer first admissions occurred to women aged between 45 and 54, than to those aged between 20 and 24, 25 and 34 and 35 and 44.

The myth that a woman becomes less stable psychologically in her middle years has other, more sinister implications. Those people who subscribe to this belief, either consciously or unconsciously, are diminishing women as a sex. If a menopausal woman is believed to be less efficient and have a reduced intellectual capacity, it can be argued that she should not be given an equal opportunity to compete with a man for a job or for promotion to a higher level. If the woman is not in the work force but has chosen to make her home her career, the believed deterioration in her mental balance and capacity may diminish her value as a person in the mind of her husband and family.

What is the truth of the matter? Are mental problems such as depression, anxiety and reduced mental efficiency more common in a woman's middle years?

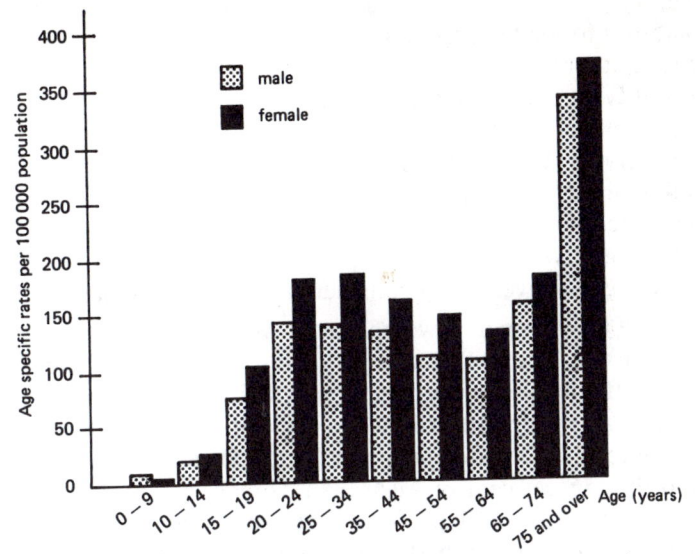

Figure 13.1: Rates of first admission to mental hospitals at various ages (Mental Health Enquiry for England, 1977)

A problem in answering this question is that studies to investigate the mental state of menopausal women have been poorly designed and often have asked the wrong questions.

These methodological problems were overcome, to some extent, in a survey conducted in Britain in 1980. One of the questions that investigators sought to answer was 'Are more women depressed in their menopausal years than at other ages?'

The survey of over 10 000 women showed that 8 out of 10 had had symptoms of depression at some time of their life; and at the time of the survey, 14 per cent were clinically depressed. Age did not seem to affect the prevalence of depression.

The survey and most others rely on a questionnaire. There are many of these, and they may give different results when administered to the same person.

A questionnaire that is used often is the General Health Questionnaire (GHQ). The version of the GHQ used to determine psychological well-being, or reduction in well-being, is based on 12 questions. The questions related to:

- inability to concentrate
- sleeplessness because of worry

- feeling of no use
- inability to make decisions
- constant strain
- inability to overcome difficulties
- no enjoyment of daily activities
- inability to face problems
- unhappiness and depression
- loss of confidence
- a feeling of worthlessness
- a feeling that everything considered resulted in unhappiness

Nearly 4000 Australian women were asked these questions in a recent survey. The women were chosen so that they were representative of the whole population. A score of 4 or more on the GHQ indicated a high or a severe psychological disturbance. A score of 2 or 3 indicated a moderate psychological disturbance. The study found that 16 per cent of Australian women had a severe psychological disturbance, 14 per cent were moderately or mildly disturbed, and 70 per cent had no psychological problems. Women in the menopausal years (aged 45 to 54) were no more psychologically disturbed than younger or older women.

Similar surveys of large numbers of women in the USA and Sweden confirm this finding. The study conducted in the USA used exacting criteria for depressive disorders and separated the depressive disorders into:

1 a major episode of depression without bereavement;
2 bereavement; and
3 any mood disorder.

In this context a mood disorder was identified if the person had at least two of the following: a poor appetite, sleep disturbance, low energy or fatigue, poor concentration and difficulty in making decisions, low self esteem and feelings of hopelessness.

Over 20 000 men and women were interviewed by trained mental health interviewers. They found that women aged 45 to 64 had fewer major depressive episodes and fewer mood disorders compared with younger women (Table 13.1).

In the Swedish study, more detailed questions were asked of women aged 38 to 54. Twenty per cent of the women complained of mental health problems (most often depression or anxiety) that affected their functioning. However, there was no increase in the proportion of women with a mental health problem in or after the

Table 13.1: Depressive disorders in women by age

| Depressive disorders | 18–24 | 25–44 | 45–64 | 65+ |
|---|---|---|---|---|
| Major episode without bereavement | 6.1 | 7.4 | 2.2 | 1.6 |
| Bereavement | 0.3 | 0.3 | 0.4 | 1.7 |
| Any mood disorder | 9.1 | 11.4 | 5.6 | 5.0 |

Data from the National Institute of Mental Health study. (USA)

menopause compared with younger women. Women who had a mental health problem before the menopause were likely to continue to have the problem after the menopause; however, the main cause of depression and anxiety were life-events. Usually, these were problems with the woman's relationship with her husband or children.

These studies confirm that there is no disease called involutional melancholia; and that depression is not more common in the menopausal years and cannot be attributed to the hormonal changes occurring at this time.

Despite these findings, some doctors continue to believe that the menopause affects the mental state of women in other ways. They suggest that in the menopausal years, a woman's memory is less effective; her concentration diminishes; she has increased difficulty in making decisions and loses her confidence. In addition it is claimed that a menopausal woman's attention span is reduced, as is her 'reaction time' in response to a question. If these observations are true, a menopausal woman may be presumed to be mentally 'inferior' to a younger woman and to men of all ages.

Are these observations true? In a British study in Oxfordshire, women and men, whose ages varied from 30 to 65, were asked a series of questions about their physical and mental health. The results were plotted for each sex and each age group (at 5 year intervals). When the psychological complaints were analysed in this way some interesting findings emerged. More women had headaches than men, but the percentage of women complaining of headaches declined from about 25 per cent in the 30 to 40 age group to 15 per cent after the age of 50. Difficulty in sleeping increased from the age of 30 in women, peaking at the age of 60, when 40 per cent of women complained. In the case of men, sleeping difficulties declined from a peak of 30 per cent at the age of 40 to 45, to 20 per cent at the age of 50 or more. More women (40 per cent) than men (25 per cent)

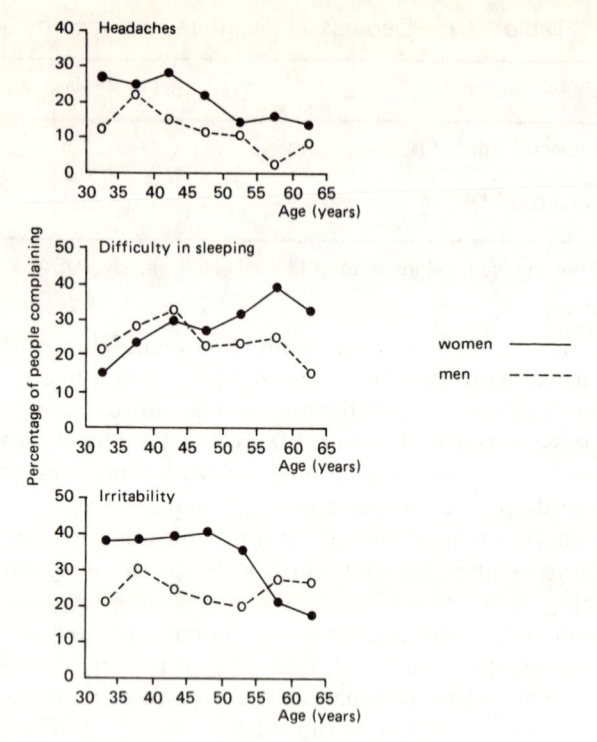

Figure 13.2: Percentage of women and men reporting headaches, difficulty in sleeping and irritability at various ages

complained of being irritable. In women the proportion complaining remained steady to the age of 40 to 50 and then declined quite rapidly, so that, by the age of 55, the proportion was similar to that of men aged 55.

From this it is clear that irritability, sleeping difficulties and headaches are not menopausal symptoms (Fig. 13.2).

It has been suggested that 'difficulty in making decisions' and 'loss in confidence' are more common in women than in men and peak after the menopause. The Oxfordshire study investigated these questions. The investigators found that at all ages from 30–35 to 60–65 women did admit to having more difficulty in making decisions than men, and also more had a loss in confidence.

When these complaints were related to the age of the woman 'difficulty in making decisions' peaked in the age group 45 to 50, at 35 per cent, and then declined from the age of 50. After the age of 55 the

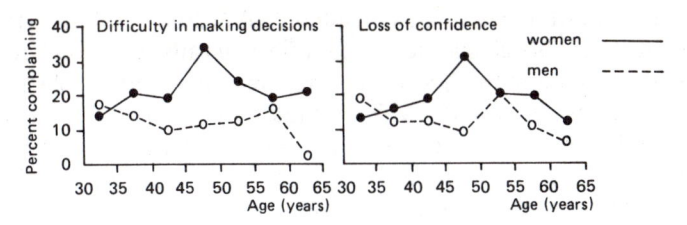

**Figure 13.3** Mental ability of men and women at various ages, as measured by the difficulty in making decisions and loss of confidence

proportion of women complaining was 20 per cent, the same as in women aged 30 to 45. The complaint of loss of confidence showed a similar pattern (Fig. 13.3). These positive findings are reassuring for menopausal women.

## Oestrogen and mood

Many menopausal women who take oestrogen say that since they have started taking the hormone they feel better and think better, and that their mood is better. Is there any truth in this? Is it possible that oestrogen has this beneficial effect?

As we have mentioned earlier, the amount of oestrogen circulating in the blood and in the tissues, including the brain, falls dramatically when the menopause occurs. Studies have shown that low blood levels of oestrogen tend to be associated with low levels of a substance in the blood called tryptophan. Tryptophan is essential for the production of a brain neurotransmitter called serotonin (also known as 5 hydroxy tryptophan). If the level in the blood of tryptophan falls so does the level of serotonin in the brain. Low brain levels of serotonin are associated with sadness, unhappiness and a depressed mood.

(It is interesting to note that many menopausal women say they feel better when they take regular exercise. Exercise taken regularly increases the brain levels of serotonin, at least in rats! If the same applies to humans, regular exercise may also benefit postmenopausal women who feel unhappy or sad.)

From this it follows that oestrogen, which increases the level of tryptophan in the blood, may also increase the levels of serotonin in the brain, and the sadness and depressed mood may be relieved, to be replaced by a feeling of well being. Oestrogen may even act as a 'mental tonic', as has been claimed.

Another matter has to be considered. A woman suffering from frequent severe hot flushes and insomnia generally feels 'low'. If she takes oestrogen and the hot flushes are controlled and she sleeps all night, she feels better and is able to think more clearly. Her mood is elevated. From this it follows that the improved mood experienced by many menopausal women taking oestrogen may be because their troublesome symptoms have been relieved.

But what about a postmenopausal woman who has no menopausal symptoms? Does her mood improve if she takes oestrogen? Apparently it does. A carefully designed study, conducted in California in 1991, showed that oestrogen taken by menopausal women who have no symptoms leads to a feeling of well-being, and an improved mood, but it does not act as a 'mental tonic'. This finding is supported by an earlier study made in Belgium, where menopausal nuns living in a closed convent were asked to take either oestrogen tablets or an identical, inert pill, without knowing which they were taking, to determine if the oestrogen pills had a mental tonic effect. Psychological tests made at the end of the study failed to find any difference in memory or in mental capacity between the two treatments. It was concluded that oestrogen did not have a mental tonic effect.

It seems unlikely that oestrogen has a mental tonic effect but it does improve a menopausal woman's quality of life, her mood and her feeling of well being, even when she has no menopausal symptoms. This is a positive finding for women.

## FATIGUE

A number of women in their middle years and especially after the menopause, complain of 'always feeling tired'. The fatigue may be due to unhappiness caused by an unsatisfactory relationship or concern about children, finances or employment. The woman hides her misery by 'somatizing' it, so that it appears as a physical disorder. Women who are in the menopausal years may feel fatigued constantly, perhaps because of somatization or because of hot flushes occurring at night, which lead to sweating. This in turn may cause insomnia with the result that the woman is tired the next day.

If a woman is constantly tired she may wish to consult a doctor who will try to find out if the problem is one of somatization or if it is due to hormone deficiency. The investigation is helped if the doctor is able to communicate well with the woman and if she is able to talk to her or him openly and frankly. If the fatigue is considered due to the oestrogen deficiency and hormone replacement treatment fails to relieve it, some studies have shown that injections of testosterone, the male hormone, help.

## SLEEP DISTURBANCES — INSOMNIA

Insomnia affects about 1 woman in 3 from time to time, and increases in prevalence as a woman grows older. Serious insomnia is reported by 1 woman in 6 and may be associated with emotional upset, psychiatric complaints or a history of alcohol or substance abuse.

Many menopausal women report sleep disturbance, which may occur during the time when the woman is having hot flushes. If these occur during the night, the woman may wake up sweating and be unable to go back to sleep. If the woman chooses to take hormone replacement, the hot flushes and the insomnia cease.

Menopausal women who do not have nocturnal hot flushes may also find that they are unable to sleep, or that they keep waking up during the night. Sleep may be disturbed because of emotional upset, or unfamiliar surroundings, or because of pain or feelings of depression. Drugs may also cause insomnia, such as some medications or excessive amounts of coffee or tea taken in the evening. It is important to realize, however, that there is no fixed 'normal' amount of sleep. Some people need 10 hours of sleep at night, others feel and perform well on 3 hours. In general, as people grow older they need less sleep and wake more frequently during the night. Older people often 'catnap' during the day, or doze in a chair in the evening. A person's perception of how much he or she sleeps may be inaccurate, and careful studies have shown that a person may be convinced that he or she has not slept all night, when in fact there have been long periods of sleep. Lack of sleep is not a problem in itself and will not in itself affect a person's health — the important thing is to discover what has produced the insomnia and then correct it.

Different people have different patterns of insomnia. For example, some people find it difficult to go to sleep but once they are asleep have no problems. Other people go to sleep easily but wake up early, feeling uncomfortable. Other people wake in the middle of the night for long periods.

How can insomnia be managed? Far too many people resort to sleeping pills, which become less effective after a time so that the

**Table 13.2:** How to help you sleep at night

* Avoid dozing during the day
* Avoid stimulants such as tea or coffee in the late evening
* Avoid alcohol beverages in the late evening
* Alcohol is a sedative and may help you to fall asleep but you may find that you wake up early in the morning
* If you find that a glass of warm milk helps you relax, then take it
* Try to deal with any problems during the day
* Spend at least one hour before going to bed, relaxing and becoming calm
* Remember that insomnia is not a disease in itself; it is the result of something else that should be treated first. Sleeping pills taken for *short periods* help to tide you over while your doctor finds out the cause of your insomnia. But if you take them for longer periods, you will find that they only help you sleep if you increase the dose, and after a while you may find it hard to give them up. If you have been taking sleeping pills for a long time, you will need to give them up, and you must realize that you may get 'withdrawal' symptoms (particularly insomnia), which can go on for weeks.

---

dose is increased. Sleeping pills (or hypnotics) are useful for brief periods to restore 'normal' patterns of sleep, but if they are taken for longer periods and then stopped, a 'withdrawal' period follows, which may last for up to 3 weeks, during which marked insomnia occurs.

Because of these problems, most women who have insomnia should first try changing some habits which may interfere with sleep (Table 13.2), before seeking sleeping pills. If the insomnia is severe and persists after changing these behaviours, sleeping pills will help. The cause of the insomnia should be taken into account in choosing a sleeping pill. For example, the benzodiazipines (Valium and similar drugs) should never be used by a woman who is depressed or is a chronic alcoholic. Recent research shows that the barbiturates and the long acting benzodiazopines (such as Valium) should not be prescribed for insomnia.

Current guidelines for doctors say that patients should not take sleeping pills for more than 2 to 4 weeks of continual use, and that short-acting sleeping pills are to be preferred. These include temazepam (Euhypnos, Normison, 20 mg); flunitrazepam (Rohypnol, 2 mg); flurazepam (Dalmane, 30 mg); nitrazepam (Mogadon, Dormicum, 10 mg). If the woman is elderly or debilitated the dose should be halved.

# 14

# SEXUALITY DURING A WOMAN'S MIDDLE YEARS

Perhaps the most useful statement about sexuality during a woman's middle years and particularly after the menopause is that although some women show a decline in their sexual desire, and in their sexual activity and sexual response with advancing age, the sexual response of an individual is unpredictable and a great variation occurs between individuals.

The human sexual response has two main parts. The first is sexual desire or sexual interest. It means that a person is sexually attracted to another person and may or may not attempt to make closer contact. If she or he does, he or she expects to become sexually aroused, in other words, has entered the second part of the sexual response. Sexual arousal may lead to sexual intercourse, to oral sex or to digital sex and, when continued, usually is climaxed by orgasm.

The frequency of sexual intercourse or of orgasm is usually taken as the measure of sexual response, but there are obvious problems in using either of these. For example, some women (and fewer men) only reach orgasm occasionally or never. As well, the ability to reach orgasm may change in frequency at different times. If the woman believes that the man should always initiate sex, the frequency of sexual intercourse may fall because the man has lost interest or appears to have lost interest.

In a study made in Sweden, about 21 per cent of women investigated had an absent or weak interest in sex after the age of 35. By the age of 54, the proportion having a weak sexual interest had increased to 52 per cent. Another Swedish investigation confirmed the finding that a woman's sexual desire tended to decline as she grew older. Out of 3000 women born in 1921, 900 were selected at random. They were interviewed when they were aged 61 to 63. One in every three said that she had lost her interest in sexual relationships.

By contrast, studies in the USA of over 20000 women aged 50 or more showed that over 90 per cent were sexually active in their 50s; over 80 per cent in their 60s and 65 per cent of the women over the age of 70 were still sexually active.

Many of the women who were not sexually active had no sexual partner, their partner was ill, or one of the couple had a medical problem. It is clear from these studies that there is as wide an individual variation in sexual desire and sexual activity in the years after the menopause, as there is in the years before the menopause.

The studies also suggest that certain women are more likely to have continued sexual interest and enjoyment into old age:

- Women who enjoyed sex in their younger years tended to enjoy sex during their middle years.
- Women who had better education, were of a higher social class and were more independent, enjoyed sex more than women of working class backgrounds. A reason for this difference may be that the working class woman had devoted her energies to looking after the home, to rearing the family and to working in a paid job. Her expectation of sexual enjoyment may have been small, particularly if her husband did not feel it his responsibility to arouse the woman sexually. It is possible that some of the women believed the myth that the sexual response either slows down or ceases when a woman reaches the menopause. It is also possible that better educated women felt more comfortable in telling a man about their sexual needs and helping him understand how he may meet them.
- Women who had episodes of depression during their reproductive years, and had a low self-esteem, were more likely to be less sexually interested or responsive in their middle years.
- Women who believed that their sexual role is one of relative passivity may experience a decline in their sexuality because they lack a man's opportunity to experience a sexual encounter.
- The husband's sexual response was a factor that must be considered. If the man was less sexually interested and had less sexual arousal, it is likely that the woman would experience sex less. The decline noted in the middle years may be as much to do with the husband's diminished interest as with the wife's.

These findings suggest that the sexual response during the later middle years is mediated by social, interpersonal or psychological events rather than being dependent on the reduced levels of the sex hormones in postmenopausal women. It is obvious that if a woman has severe hot flushes or a dry, uncomfortable vagina, due to a lack of circulating oestrogen, she is likely neither to desire sexual intercourse nor to enjoy it if it takes place. Oestrogen treatment will improve the woman's sex life by relieving the symptoms, but the improvement is not due to a direct effect of oestrogen on her sexual desire or arousal. This is demonstrated by the finding that some women who have a dry, uncomfortable vagina enjoy cuddling and may enjoy pleasuring their partner sexually although they do not want vaginal penetration because of the discomfort.

There is some evidence in some women that the reduced level of sexual desire may be related to a fall in the level of the male hormone, testosterone, in their blood and brain. In laboratory animals, a lack of testosterone is associated with a decreased sexual response. Some studies have shown that some postmenopausal women who have higher blood level of testosterone have an increased sexual desire, but this is of less importance than a good relationship with her partner.

The animal findings have persuaded some doctors to offer injections of testosterone to postmenopausal women who have a reduced sexual desire or response. The results of investigations reported since 1975 are contradictory. There is no consensus among experts that testosterone injections increase a postmenopausal woman's sexual desire or arousal.

Because of the controversy, a sensible approach a woman may choose to take is to see if oestrogen alone improves her sexual desire (by relieving hot flushes and vaginal symptoms), and if it does not, to have an injection of testosterone (50 mg), every 3 to 6 months, in addition.

## HOW TO IMPROVE SEXUAL RELATIONSHIPS

The sexual problems that affect women in the middle years are no different from those affecting younger women, with one exception. This is the problem of painful intercourse. Painful intercourse may occur at all ages for a variety of reasons, but in menopausal and postmenopausal women it may be due to a lack of oestrogen. Oestrogen lack leads to a thinner vaginal lining, to a burning pain or discomfort in the vagina and to painful intercourse. The treatment is to give oestrogen, as was discussed on page 56.

However, it may be important for the couple to explore the relationship as well.

Lack of sexual desire, lack of sexual arousal and failure to reach orgasm are due, usually, to conflict in the couple's relationships. The underlying factors may be that the couple have stopped talking to each other, and that neither partner is able to tell the other of her or his sexual needs or feelings. The woman may see her husband as fat, ageing or drinking too much. He may see her body as flabby and ageing and may compare it adversely with the bodies of the models and actresses he sees on television or in videos. The woman may sense this and lose her confidence, becoming depressed. She may no longer feel she has any worth to her husband. She may have become bored with the way her husband makes love, particularly if she has been brought up to believe that the man is always the initiator.

The first way to improve matters is for the couple to try to talk to each other about their relationship. It may help if first they both have a medical check-up to make sure that the problem is not an underlying undiscovered illness. If the woman is able to talk about her sexual desires, her needs and her feelings, and her husband is able to reciprocate, the problem may be resolved. If they always make love in exactly the same way, they may agree to try something more innovative. If the man believes that unless his wife reaches orgasm while he thrusts inside her she is frigid, he needs to reassess this belief. It is wrong. Fewer than half of all women reach orgasm in this way. To help his wife reach orgasm, she may ask her partner to stimulate her clitoris, at her direction, or she may find she reaches orgasm by masturbating.

The second way to improve her sexual enjoyment is for her to seek sexual counselling from a doctor, a psychologist or a psychiatrist and to induce her husband to come with her for some of the sessions at least.

Sexuality includes cuddling, touching and holding as well as sexual intercourse. Sexuality includes feeling that you are of value to your partner and he values you. And this is of considerable importance to a woman in her middle years.

# BIBLIOGRAPHY

Only key references are given.

## Chapter 2  A WOMAN'S REPRODUCTIVE ORGANS
**The anatomy of the genital tract and the physiology of menstruation**
Llewellyn-Jones D, *Fundamentals of Obstetrics and Gynaecology*, Vol 2: Gynaecology. 5th edn, London, Faber, 1990.

## Chapter 3  A WOMAN IN HER FORTIES
**Fertility and contraception**
Bowen-Simpkins C, in *Contraception — Science and Practise*. Eds: Filshie M, Guillebaud J, London, Butterworth, 1989, 224–38; Navot D, *Lancet* 1991, 337, 1375.
**Premenstrual syndrome**
Llewellyn-Jones D et al., *New Ethicals*, Nov 1990, 85–93.
**Endometrial ablation**
Magos A, *Lancet* 1991, 337, 1074–8, and correspondence.

## Chapter 4  HEALTHY EATING IN THE MIDDLE YEARS
**General**
Better Health Commission: *Looking Forward to Better Health*, vol. 2: Towards Better Nutrition for Australia, Canberra, AGPS, 1987; Llewellyn-Jones D, Abraham S, *Eating Disorders — The Facts*. 3rd edn., Oxford, Oxford University Press, 1992, Llewellyn — Jones D, Everybody Oxford, Oxford University Press, 1992.

## Chapter 5  THE MENOPAUSE
**Perceptions of menopausal symptoms in various cultures**
Payer L, in *A Portrait of the Menopause*. Eds: Burger H, Boulet M, Carnforth, Parthenon, 1991, 3–22; Avis N E and McKinley S, *Maturitas* 1991, 10, 65–79; Lock M, *Lancet* 1991, 337, 1270–2.

## Chapter 6  PSYCHOLOGICAL CHANGES IN THE MENOPAUSAL YEARS

**Life stress and menopausal symptoms**
Greene J G and Cooke J, *Brit J Psychiat* 1986, 136, 486–91; Poht D E, La Rocca S A, *Psych Medicine* 1980, 42, 335–45; Ballinger S E. *Maturitas* 1985, 7, 315–27.

**Effect of oestrogen treatment on mood**
Ditkoff E et al., *Obstet Gynec* 1991, 78, 991–5.

## Chapter 7  PHYSICAL SYMPTOMS IN THE MENOPAUSAL YEARS

**Proportion of menopausal women who have 'distressing' symptoms**
Thompson B et al., *J Biosocial Sci* 1973, 5, 71–82; James C E, *Brit J Obst and Gynaec* 1984, 91, 56–62; Bungay G J et al. (Oxfordshire Study): *Brit Med J* 1980, 281, 181–84; (Swedish studies) Person T et al., *Acta Obst Gynaec Scand* 1983, 62, 289–96; 1984, 63, 257–70; Hagstad A and Jansen P O, *Acta Obst Gynaec Scand* Supp 134, 1986, 59–65; Oldenhave A, in *Abst 6th Int. Congress on Menopause*. Abst 093. Carnforth, Parthenon, 1990.

## Chapter 8  HOW TO MANAGE THE MENOPAUSE

**Attitudes to and perceptions of the menopause**
See references to Chapter 5.

**Hormone replacement treatment; how prescribed**

**Progestogen every 3rd month**
Kemp J, *ANZ J Obst Gynaec* 1989, 26, 66–9.

**Combined continuous oestrogen and progestogen**
Christiansen C, Riis B J, *Brit J Obst Gynaec* 1990, 87, 1087–92.

**Livial**
Tax L et al., *Maturitas* 1987, 9, supp 1.

**Transdermal oestrogen**
Miller-Bass K, *Fert Steril* 1990, 53, 961–74.

**Implants**
Brincat M et al., *Lancet* 1984, 1, 16–19.

**Breast cancer and HRT**
See chapter 9 for references.

**Why do all postmenopausal women not take HRT?**
Avis N E et al., *Ann NY Acad Sci* 1990, 592, 228–38; Hahn R G, *Amer J Obst Gynec* 1989, 161, 1854–8; Nachtigall L E, *Obstet Gynec* 1990, Supp 77s–80s; Wilkes H C et al., *Brit Med J* 1991, 302, 1317–20.

**Oestrogen metabolism**
Casey M L and MacDonald P, *The Menopause*, Buchsbaum H J (ed), New York, Springer-Verlag, 1983, 1–23; Fishman J and Matucci C P, 'New Concepts of Oestrogen Activity', *Menopause and Postmenopause*, Pasetto N (ed), Lancaster, MTP, 1980.

## Chapter 9  THE SIDE-EFFECTS OF HORMONAL TREATMENT
**Cancer of the endometrium**
Gunn A D in *A Portrait of the Menopause*. Eds: Burger H, Boulet M, Carnforth, Parthenon, 1991.
**Cancer of the breast**
Conference report on the menopause. *Obstet Gynec* 1990, Supp 75, 815–38; Hulka B S et al., *Ca-A Cancer J* 1991, 40, 289–96; Dupont W D et al., *Arch Int Med* 1991, 151, 67–72.


## Chapter 10  OSTEOPOROSIS
**General review**
Llewellyn-Jones D, in *Portrait of the Menopause*. Eds: Burger H, Boulet M, Carnforth, Parthenon, 1991, 83–103.
**Fractures and ageing**
Grisso J A, *New Eng J Med* 1991, 324, 1326–32; Porter R W, *Brit Med J* 1990, 301, 638–41; Winner S J, *Brit Med J* 1989, 298, 1486–88.
**Prevalence of osteoporosis**
Michell D, *Amer J Obst Gynec* 1989, 161, 1851–68.
**Prophylaxis and treatment**
Consensus Development Report *Amer J Med* 1991, 90, 107–110.


## Chapter 11  THE MIDDLE YEARS AND THE BODY SYSTEMS
**Cardiovascular disease**
**Prevention of heart attacks**
Bush T L et al., *Circulation* 1987, 75, 259–74; Sitruk-Ware P, *Maturitas* 1989, 11, 259–74; Mathews K A, *New Eng Med J* 1989, 321, 641–5.
**Risk of death from coronary heart disease in women**
Castelli W D, *Amer J Obst Gynec* 1988, 158, 1552–60.
**HRT and cardiovascular system**
Ginsburg J in *Portrait of the Menopause*. Eds: Burger H, Boulet M, Carnforth, Pergamon, 1991, 45–66.
**Urinary tract. Incontinence and ageing**
Mollander W et al., *Maturitas* 1990, 12, 51–60.
**Breasts. Self examination**
Material courtesy Anti-cancer Council of Victoria.
**Value of mammography screening**
UK Trial: Early Detection of Brest Cancer British Med J 1992; 304:346.


## Chapter 12  A WOMAN'S SKIN IN HER MIDDLE YEARS
Bolognia J L, *Maturitas* 1989, 11, 295–304.

## Chapter 13 THE MIND IN A WOMAN'S MIDDLE YEARS

**Prevalence of psychiatric disorders**
Gath D et al. *Brit Med J* 1987, 294, 213–18; Gath D, Editorial, *Brit Med J* 1990, 300, 1287–8; Halstrom T et al., *Acta Obst Gynaec Scand* 1985, Supp 130, 13–15.

**Insomnia**
Gillin C, *New Eng J Med* 1991, 324, 1735–65.

## Chapter 14 SEXUALITY DURING A WOMAN'S MIDDLE YEARS

**General**
Brecher E M, *Love, Sex and Aging.* Boston, Little Brown, 1984; Bachmann G A, *Maturitas* 1991, 13, 41–50.

**Testosterone implants to increase libido**
Of value: Burger H, *Brit Med J* 1987, 294, 936–7. No value: Dow M G T *Brit J Obst Gynaec* 1983, 90, 361–6; Bachman H, *Maturitas* 1985, 7, 211–16.

# GLOSSARY

**Androgens**   male sex hormones. These include testosterone.

**Artificial menopause**   The cessation of a woman's menstrual period following surgical removal of her ovaries or radiation to her ovaries, and if not treated she may develop menopausal symptoms.

**Body mass index (BMI)**   An index of the body weight to determine if the person is underweight, if weight is in the normal range, or if the person is overweight or obese. The index is calculated using the following formula:

$$\frac{\text{Weight in kilograms}}{\text{Height in metres} \times \text{height in metres}}$$

**Cholesterol**   An important constituent of animal fats (lipids) which is involved in the development of narrowing (atherosis) of the arteries of the heart. In the body, cholesterol links with lipoproteins to be carried in the blood. Cholesterol is linked with several of the lipoprotein fractions, which have different densities. They are named high-density lipoprotein (HDL), low-density lipoprotein (LDL) and very-low-density lipoprotein (VLDL). The higher the level of the LDL–cholesterol fraction in the blood, the greater is the risk of a heart attack.

**Climacteric**   (Sometimes referred to as 'perimenopause') The period of hormonal and psychological adjustment around the time of the menopause. The word is no longer in fashion and menopause is used in its place. If the term 'menopause' is used accurately it means the permanent cessation of menstruation, not the years around the event.

**Collagen**   The white substance that forms fibres in the connective tissues, cartilege and bone. On boiling, it turns into gelatin.

**Cortical layer of bone**   The compressed outer layer of true bone. Also called cortical or compact bone.

**Cystitis**   Infection of the urinary bladder.

**Dermis**   The layer of the skin between the outside layer (the epidermis) and the connective tissue. The dermis contains hair follicles, sweat glands and blood vessels.

**Endometrium**   The inner layer of the uterus, which contains the uterine glands.

**Endometriosis**  The growth of endometrium in the pelvis, for example, on an ovary or in the Pouch of Douglas. It is thought that fragments of the endometrium reach the pelvic cavity via the fallopain tubes during menstruation.

**Epidermis**  The outer layer of the skin.

**Follicle stimulating hormone**  One of the hormones secreted by the pituitary gland, which stimulates the growth of a number of egg cells in the ovary each month during a woman's reproductive years. It is also known as FSH. FSH stimulates the cells that surround the egg to secrete oestrogen.

**Labia**  The 'lips' that surround the entrance to the vagina. The outer lips (labia majora) are filled with fatty tissue and have hair on the outer surface; the inner lips (labia minora) are thin and have no hair on them.

**Luteinizing hormone (LH)**  The second of the pituitary hormones that are involved in releasing an ovum (egg) each month during the reproductive years. LH then acts on the cell nest from which the egg escaped and converts it into a 'yellow body'. The yellow body (corpus luteum) secretes oestrogen and progesterone.

**Mammography**  The technique of making an X-ray picture of the breasts; it uses a very small, and safe quantity of radiation. The picture is called a mammogram.

**Oestrogen**  The main female sex hormone.

**Osteoporosis**  The loss of bone tissue and of calcium, which renders the bone brittle and more likely to fracture.

**Perimenopause**  *See* Climacteric.

**Periosteum**  The thin, transparent tissue that covers bone.

**Progesterone**  The second of the female sex hormones.

**Progestogens**  Progesterone-like substances produced in a laboratory. In the body they have many of the effects of the natural hormone progesterone, but unlike it, they are effective if taken by mouth.

**Quetelet Index**  Another name for the body mass index, so called after the scientist who first used it.

**Trabecular bone**  The inner part of the long bones, and most of the vertebral bones of the spine. It is made up of a complicated honeycomb of bony tissue.

**Vulva**  A woman's external genitals.

# INDEX

Ageing
  bone changes during  104
  fractures and  95–97, 109–111
  height changes in  94–95, 110
  mental health and  155–162
artificial menopause, see menopause, artificial

biopsy, breast
  endometrium  89–90
bleeding
  postmenopausal  133
  withdrawal  70, 73, 81
blood pressure, high  92, 127, 128
body mass index (BMI)  39
bone
  calcium in formation of  101
  changes with ageing  92–95, 104–106
  compact layer, see bone, cortical
  cortical  98
  density measurement  115
  description of  97–101
  dynamism of  97
  exercise and  117
  fractures of  95–97, 109–111
  oestrogen and  103
  remodelling of  97
  spongy bone, see bone, trabecular
  structure of  98–99
  trabecular  98
breasts
  cancer, see cancer, breast
  changes
    menstrual cycle during  12
    menopause, after  12, 137
  examination of  142–143
  mammography of  143–145
  self-examination (BSE) of  137–142

body image  2

caffeine intake  63, 87
calciferol, see hormones, calciferol
calcitonin, see hormones, calcitonin
calcium
  and bone  94, 101–104, 112–114
  diet in  37–38
  osteoporosis in  101–104, 112–114, 121
cancer
  breast  80, 81, 90
  cervix  9
  endometrium  27, 65, 81, 88, 134
  ovary  135
cardiovascular disease  91, 122–128
  reducing risk of  128
cervix, uterine
  description of  9
  cancer of  9
cholesterol  125
cigarette smoking  64
civilization, diseases of  36
climacteric  43
Climen  66
clitoris  5
condom  22
contraception
  condom  22
  diaphragm  22
  Pill, the  20
  tubal sterilization  20
  vasectomy  20
collagen
  bone in  99
  skin in  149
cortical bone, see bone, cortical
curettage  27, 133

danazol 28, 30
Deca Durabolin 120
depression 158
desogestrel 71
diaphragm, vaginal 22
Didronel 119
diet
  principles of 33–38
  calcium in 37
  fats in 34, 125
  fibre in 36–37
  habits, bad 38
  healthy 33
  sugar in 35
  weight reducing 40–42
Dowager's hump 96, 109
Duphaston 71
dydrogesterone 71

endometrium
  biopsy of 28, 89, 133
  cancer of 27, 65, 81, 88, 134
  oestrogens and 67
  progestogens and 69
Estace 66
Estraderm 66
Estigen 66
ethinyl oestradiol 65
etidronate 117, 119
exercise 61, 117, 161
  osteoporosis for 117
  relaxation 61

Fallopian tubes 10
fatigue 162
fat in diet 34
Feminone 66
fertility, decline after 40 19
fibre in diet 36–37
fibroids 28
flashes, hot, *see* flushes, hot
fluoride for osteoporosis 117, 120
flushes, hot 53–56
follicle stimulating hormone, *see*
  hormones, follicle stimulating
fractures, bone, *see* bone, fractures of
FSH, *see* hormones, follicle stimulating

gall bladder disease 92
General Health Questionnaire 157
genital organs 5–11
  changes after menopause 11–12
  changes in with age 11–12
genitals

external 4–7
internal 7–11
Gestrinone 28

hair, oestrogen and 154
Harmogen 66
heart disease 122–128
height, decrease in with ageing 95–97
hip fractures 95
hormonal replacement treatment
  (therapy) 26, 64–82
  contraindications to 80
  effectiveness of 77
  investigations before use 79
  misconceptions about 84
  principles of 65, 81
  side-effects of 60–4
  regimens of 72–79
  resistance to using 83
  testosterone in 77
hot flushes (flashes), *see* flushes, hot
hormones
  calcitonin 117, 119
  calcitriol 120
  changes before menopause 16
  changes after menopause 17
  follicle stimulating 12, 17
  gonadotrophic releasing 14–15
  luteinizing 13
  oestrogen 13, 64–77, 114, 118, 127
  parathyroid 103
  progesterone 15
  progestogens 69–72, 92
  testosterone 18, 27, 117, 167
  thyroid 145
hymen 6
hysterectomy 29, 72, 81
  effects of 29
  incidence of 29
  myths about 29
  sex after 29
hysteroscopy 27

implants
  oestrogen 76, 78
  testosterone 167
incontinence, urinary 129–133
  coping with 131
  diagnosis of 131–132
  exercises in 132
  vaginal cones in 132
  varieties of 130
insomnia 63, 159, 163–164
intrauterine device (IUD) 31

# INDEX

'involutional melancholia' 156

Kliogest 66
Kolpon pessaries 66

labia
    majora 4
    minora 5
levonorgestrel 70, 71
life expectancy 46
lipids (in blood) 84, 125–126
lipoproteins 125–126
Livial 65, 71, 74
luteinizing hormone (LH) *see* hormones, luteinizing
Lynoral 66

mammography 143–145
medroxyprogesterone (Provera) 28, 70, 71, 80, 82
menopause
    age of 45
    approach to 60, 83–84
    'artificial' 46
    breasts and 12, 137
    coping with 50
    cultural views of 43–45
    definition of 43
    doctors' views of 46–48
    exercise during 61
    hot flushes during 54–56
    hormonal changes during 16–18
    hormonal treatment of 64–82
    non-hormonal treatment of 82
    physical
        symptoms of 52–56
        management of 64–82
    psychological
        symptoms of 58–59
        management of 57–64
    premature 45
    urinary symptoms during 129
    vaginal symptoms during 56
    vasomotor symptoms during 54–56
menstruation
    control of 12–16
    heavy 27
    hormone treatment for 28
    hysterectomy for 29–30
    irregular 26–27
    IUD in 31
mental health in middle years 155–162
moisturizers 151–153

mood disorders 158, 161
myoma 27

nandrolone decanoate 120
night sweats 54
norethisterone 29, 69, 71, 82
norgestimate 70

obesity 32, 38–42, 124
    abdominal 124
    complications of 32, 39–40
    heart disease and 124
    treatment of 40–42
oestradiol 85
oestriol 87
oestrogens
    blood pressure and 92
    cancer and 88–92
    cardiovascular disease and 126–127
    conjugated equine oestrogens 66, 85
    estropipate (ogen) 66, 86
    hair and 154
    heart disease and 126–127
    injection of 76
    implant of 76, 78
    liver function and 68, 85
    menopause in 65
    menstrual cycle in 13
    metabolism of 67, 85
    micronized 72
    misconceptions about 84
    mood and 161
    'natural' 65, 67, 68, 86
    oestriol 66, 87
    oestradiol valerate 66, 87
    oral 86
    osteoporosis and 114, 118
    percutaneous and 75
    side-effects of 88–93
    skin and 150
    synthetic 65
    transdermal 74
    vaginal 74
    varieties of 66, 86
Ogen 66
osteoporosis
    bone density screening in 115
    caffeine intake and 107
    calcitonin in 117, 119
    calcitriol in 120
    calcium in 94, 101–104, 112–114, 121

'causes' of 106–107
costs of 108
definition of 94
development of 94
exercise and 117
fractures in 95–97, 109–111
oestrogens in 103, 106, 114, 115, 118
progestogens in 114
prevention of 112–116
smoking and 89
symptoms of 108
treatment of 118–121
ovarian failure, premature 45
ovaries 10
overweight 32, 124
Ovestin 66
oviducts (Fallopian tubes) 10
ovulation 13

Pap smear 9, 63, 134
pelvic floor exercises 132
perimenopause 48–50
  problems during 48
perineum 5
periosteum 98
Pill, the 20
postmenopausal bleeding 133
Premarin 66, 69
premenstrual syndrome 24
Prempak 69
Primolut-N 28, 69, 71
progesterone, *see* hormones, progesterone
progestogens 69–72
  treatment using 28
  side-effects of 71, 92
Progynova 66
Provera 28, 69, 71, 80, 82

Relaxation exercises 26, 61–62

sex hormones, *see* hormones
sexual intercourse, painful 56, 65
sexual problems 2, 166–168
sexual relations
  in later years 165–167
  improving 167–168
sexual response 166
sexuality
  in middle years 165–167
  testosterone and 167

skin
  changes with ageing 149–150
  collagen in 149
  description of 147–148
  'foods' 151–153
  moisturizers and 151–153
  oestrogens and 150
  photoaged 153
sleeping pills 164
smoking 64
stroke 128
sugar, diet in 35
sweats 54–56

thyroid disease 145
tibolone 66
testosterone, *see* hormones, testosterone
thrombosis, venous 91
trabecular bone, *see* bone, trabecular
transdermal oestrogen, *see* oestrogen, transdermal
tubal ligation 20

ultrasound, for diagnosis 27
urinary incontinence, *see* incontinence, urinary
uterine cervix, *see* cervix, uterine
Uterogestan 66
uterus, description 9

vagina 7–9, 56
vaginal oestrogen 56, 65
vaginal smears 56
vaginal symptoms in menopause
  burning 56, 65
  discomfort 56, 65
  pain 56, 65
vasectomy 20
vasomotor symptoms 54
venous thrombosis, *see* thrombosis, venous
vitamins in diet 38
vitamin $D_3$ 103
vulva (external genitals) 4

'withdrawal bleed' 70, 73
weight gain with ageing 32–33, 63
weight reducing diet 40–42
work outside home 2
wrinkles 149